Surgery Junkies

Wellness and Pathology in Cosmetic Culture

Victoria Pitts-Taylor

Rutgers University Press

New Brunswick, New Jersey, and London

Library of Congress Cataloging-in-Publication Data

Pitts-Taylor, Victoria.
  Surgery junkies : wellness and pathology in cosmetic culture /
Victoria Pitts-Taylor.
    p. cm.
  Includes bibliographical references and index.
  ISBN-13: 978-0-8135-4047-4 (hardcover : alk. paper)
  ISBN-13: 978-0-8135-4048-1 (pbk. : alk. paper)
  1. Surgery, Plastic—Psychological aspects.   2. Surgery, Plastic—
Social aspects.   I. Title.
  [DNLM: 1. Cosmetic Techniques—psychology.   2. Reconstruc-
tive Surgical Procedures—psychology.   3. Behavior, Addictive.
WO 600 P692s 2007]
  RD119.P52 2007
  617.9'520973—dc22   2006025456

A British Cataloging-in-Publication record for this book is available
from the British Library

Manufactured in the United States of America

To Gregory Warwick Taylor, MD, PhD,
with deepest gratitude and affection

Contents

Acknowledgments

I am very grateful to all of the people who agreed to be interviewed for this book. There are also many other people who need to be thanked. They include my colleagues and friends at Queens College and the Graduate Center, City University of New York: Patricia Clough, Deidre Conlon, Paisley Currah, Mitch Duneier, Hester Eisenstein, Harry Levine, Milt Mankoff, Lisa Jean Moore, Robin Rogers-Dillon, Lauren Seiler, Dean Savage, and Charlie Smith. For their research assistance, I thank Joli Brown, Danielle Wellington and Maria Russell. At Brandeis University, Peter Conrad organized a lecture that provided the first audience for my work on surgery addiction. I also want to thank Arthur Frank, who offered invaluable advice and feedback. Other people who gave various kinds of help include Stefan Timmermans, Meredith Jones, Jon Mowitt, Ed Lenert, Brenda Weber, Debra Gimlin, Abigail Brooks, the Honorable Mark Taylor, Chris and Jana Julka, and Nikki Sullivan. In addition, I thank my graduate students in the 2005 Sociology of Bodies Seminar at CUNY Graduate Center for stimulating and challenging my thinking.

At the University of California Santa Cruz, I thank Helene Moglen and Nancy Chen of the Institute for Advanced Feminist Research for organizing the 2005 conference on "Bodies in the Making" and inviting me to give the address.

Much of chapter 1 is based on my talk there, which was first published in the IAFR Feminist Provocations series. At the Biomedical Ethics Unit/Faculty of Medicine of McGill University, Montreal, Leigh Turner organized the "Surgical Solutions" conference in 2006, which brought together ten scholars writing on cosmetic surgery. I thank him and all of the participants for helping me further my thinking on this topic. At Rutgers University Press, Kristi Long gave me her trust and support, and Adi Hovav, my editor, offered help, guidance, and patience. I thank Joe Rollins for assisting with chapter 5, as well for taking me to see Eve Ensler's *The Good Body*, which I discuss in chapter 3, for attending the Bodies conference with me and, most important, for his enduring and invaluable friendship for the past eight years.

Personal life feeds intellectual life. I thank my friends and family for the various ways in which they supported me personally during the years of this writing and research. In addition to those already mentioned, they include Maureen O'Sullivan, who has been a dear friend, and Elizabeth Wood, who has been an important part of my life for over a decade. I am grateful to my parents for their help and encouragement. I thank Milan Ferencei for his encouragement and humor. My sisters, Jennifer Anna Gosetti-Ferencei and Angela Gosetti-Murray John, are inspirations to me in many ways, and I must acknowledge all of their guidance over the years, which has been considerable. I also thank Jennifer for her critique of chapter 3. I am lucky to have such intellectually powerful sisters, and even luckier to have their abiding friendship and enthusiastic support of my work and life.

Finally, and most especially, I am indebted to Gregory Warwick Taylor, MD, PhD, for more than I can possibly list, but including: our stimulating conversations about medicine and other bodily subjects, his kind interest and ongoing support of my work, his feedback on many of the chapters here, his various efforts to help me finish this volume, his brilliance in his work and dedication to his patients, his perseverance in keeping me healthy, and most especially, for making my personal life so fulfilling. I dedicate this book to him, with my deepest gratitude and affection.

Surgery Junkies

Introduction

Dr. James McCullen, a plastic and reconstructive surgeon in New England, believes that Lydia Manderson, one of his former patients, is a "cosmetic surgery junkie." Dr. McCullen is a well-regarded, board-certified plastic surgeon who once specialized in reconstructive surgery of the limbs, and now devotes much of his practice to body contouring, which includes body lifts, breast implants, and liposuction. His patient Lydia is an affluent widow who is very enthusiastic about cosmetic surgery.[1] Over several years, Dr. McCullen performed multiple surgeries on her face and body. But he has come to believe that Lydia is never satisfied; she is always seeking more beautification or rejuvenation. As he put it in an interview: "She has the money and she wants every little thing done and she's never going to stop." He believes that no matter how much surgery she gets, there will always be another part of the body she will want lifted, tucked, or transformed. Eventually, McCullen decided to end his doctor-patient relationship with Lydia. The last straw for him came when Lydia, as he put it, "went off to New York and had an arm tuck done." When she was unhappy with the resulting scars, she asked Dr. McCullen to do another surgery to fix the problem. He refused, because he no longer saw Lydia as a good patient. As he put it: "I don't see her anymore. I don't want my signature on her body."

Dr. McCullen believes that it is important for the surgeon to be discerning about his patients. "You make your reputation," he said, "as much on who you turn away as on who you operate on." But how are cosmetic surgery patients sorted? Why was Lydia Manderson considered a surgery junkie by her own surgeon? Since he had performed multiple surgeries on other patients, what made her different? What prompted Dr. McCullen to decide, after a series of procedures, that she'd had one surgery too many? Dr. McCullen worried aloud whether his patient was psychologically unwell. McCullen's assertion that she is a "junkie" means that she has a pathological addiction to cosmetic surgery. In fact, Dr. McCullen told me that he believes she may have Body Dysmorphic Disorder (BDD), a mental disorder characterized by a person's obsession about a slight or imagined flaw in her or his appearance to the point of clinically significant distress or dysfunction.

In the past twenty years, the cosmetic surgery junkie has become a social problem, identified from a variety of perspectives as representing the worst-case scenario of cosmetic surgery. The cosmetic surgery junkie might be the patient who has been turned away by the surgeon as a so-called "poor candidate" for a cosmetic procedure, or one who is considered chronically unhappy, litigious, or difficult by her surgeon. In psychiatry, she is increasingly given the diagnosis of BDD and is prescribed an antidepressant and cognitive-behavior therapy. In the media, the surgery junkie might be a celebrity who seems to have had too much cosmetic surgery or someone who has unusual taste in body modification. In the courtroom, the surgery junkie may enter as a plaintiff, arguing that she is a victim of medical malpractice. In feminist writings, surgery junkies are women who, in their desperation to adhere to the standards of beauty culture, become "surgical."[2] And for some feminist critics of cosmetic surgery, *anyone* who undergoes an elective cosmetic surgery is a victim who will eventually get hooked on surgical beautification.

The rise of public concern over cosmetic surgery excess and addiction parallels cosmetic surgery's astonishing expansion. Cosmetic modifications of the body have expanded dramatically in number, type, and scope. For instance, in theUnited States in 2005, there were nearly two million aesthetic operations—more than quadruple the number in 1984—along with over eight million nonsurgical procedures like Botox and skin resurfacing.[3] And with the vast expansion in the number of cosmetic procedures, cosmetic surgery has been democratized, with the majority of patients now in the middle class. There has also been surgical innovation, from new approaches to the face-lift to surgery on new areas of the body, such as rib removal, buttocks implants, and genital surgeries such as labiaplasty. In addition, patients getting cosmetic surgery increasingly have multiple procedures during the same operation—in 2004, for example, one-third of cosmetic surgeries involved multiple procedures. It is now ordinary for a cosmetic surgeon to package procedures, like a chin implant to go with a rhinoplasty, or a breast lift to go with a tummy tuck.[4] The market boom has encouraged many doctors to expand their practices to include cosmetic procedures. Since any licensed medical doctor, whatever his or her specialty, can perform cosmetic surgeries, all kinds of physicians, including dentists and ophthalmologists, are newly entering the cosmetic surgery market.[5] And cosmetic surgery is now culturally ubiquitous. On television, in magazines, and on the Web, there are endless discussions of cosmetic surgery, from makeover shows where participants get multiple surgeries to documentaries and celebrity gossip. Beauty and health magazines, local television news programs, and the Internet are replete with consumer information about cosmetic surgery—how to shop for a surgeon, what procedures are better than others, what the latest technology can accomplish. It is perhaps unsurprising, then, that recent studies suggest that Americans are increasingly comfortable with cosmetic surgery.[6] All of these developments point toward its normalization.

Thus, in contrast to Lydia's story, when in the midst of writing this book I decided to have my own cosmetic surgery, I found that I was a "good candidate" for such a procedure. Cosmetic surgeons I visited believed that I had the right reasons, was an acceptable age, wanted the right procedures, and had the proper attitude. I was expressing, according to the advocates of cosmetic surgery, a sense of psychological wellness by embracing surgery to improve my looks. (I underwent rhinoplasty, which reshaped my nose in the direction of normative beauty ideals.) Many of my friends and colleagues were aghast, identifying women who get cosmetic surgery as dupes of beauty culture and worrying that cosmetic surgery is addictive. Yet the surgeon who performed my operation told me that "people don't see it as a big deal anymore." Another doctor, a dermatologist who sees many Botox patients, told me that conventional fears and criticisms about cosmetic surgery are for the most part "outdated," that people are no longer ashamed of having cosmetic surgery. (In fact, he pointed out that some people now even want what he called the "plastic look" in order to show off their surgeries, as a form of conspicuous consumption.) My choice to have cosmetic surgery, in their view, was an ordinary decision made by increasing numbers of people just like me. The doctors even presented other options I might think about: my surgeon thought I might also like a chin implant, while the dermatologist recommended ble-pharoplasty (eyelid lift).

In the eyes of our cosmetic surgeons, Lydia and I are at either end of a spectrum ranging from pathological to normal, from bad to good patient. I am interested in considering the social production of this spectrum. My surgery and Lydia's have both taken place in a historical moment of social uncertainty about cosmetic surgery, in which we are managing our continued ambivalence about it while forging ahead with its unprecedented expansion. In this book, I examine the social construction of extreme cosmetic surgery, cosmetic surgery junkies, and surgery addiction, along with some of the recent manifestations of good and normal cosmetic surgery and patients. In my view, these constructions represent our attempts to socially manage the virtual explosion of cosmetic surgery in our society. I explore some of the processes by which we are deciding what kinds of surgeries, and which kinds of patients, we will socially accept and promote. What are the good and bad surgeries? What are the acceptable and unacceptable reasons for cosmetic surgery? Who are the acceptable and unacceptable patients?

The term "cosmetic surgery junkie" is often used to refer to people who have been deemed "extreme" in their use of cosmetic surgery by various actors and observers. The term is widely used, along with terms such as "plasta-holic," "surgery addict," and "obsessed cosmetic surgery patient." These terms are often used interchangeably, although in some contexts, such as the early psychiatric literature on cosmetic surgery patients, distinctions among them are made. What they share is that they stigmatize people whose surgeries are socially disturbing. In this book, I refer to junkies, addicts, and people obsessed with cosmetic surgery, but I hope it is clear that I do not use these terms to contribute to the stigmatization of people who get cosmetic surgery. Instead, I look at how people are named with these labels, and at the ways such extremes and their corresponding norms are socially determined. I examine the spectacle of extreme makeovers created in the media; the negative characterization of some cosmetic surgery patients as junkies in the media; the medicalization of cosmetic surgery addiction as Body Dysmorphic Disorder, among other diagnoses; the specter of the difficult patient for cosmetic surgeons in the clinic and the courtroom; and feminists' fears about cosmetic surgery. In tracing how these pathologies are socially constructed, I am not endorsing, but rather problematizing, their apparent meanings.

The expected feminist argument against cosmetic surgery is based on the assumption that all cosmetic surgery mutilates the body, victimizes the subject, or expresses her internal pathology. I do not begin from this viewpoint. Neither do I champion cosmetic surgery as a sign of cosmetic wellness or personal empowerment, as cosmetic surgeons and some sympathetic observers have done. Instead, I try to denaturalize the extremes and norms of cosmetic surgery, exposing their social constructedness. One of my primary aims is to show how the meanings of cosmetic surgery are being variously produced in consumer capitalism, medicine, psychiatry, and politics. In postmodern cultures our bodies have been positioned as signs of our personal, individual identities. Thus the cosmetic surgery lobbies and the television spectacles of cosmetic surgery identify important aspects of ourselves—our inner beauty and our sense of personal wellness—that are expressed in cosmetic surgery. And the psychiatric and psychotherapeutic perspectives have identified the truth of cosmetic surgery according to a diagnostic model that has historically assumed the mental pathology of cosmetic surgery patients. Many feminists have identified women's self-hatred and internalized oppression in cosmetic surgery practices. Others, like medical sociologist Kathy Davis, have argued that women are employing rational agency in their decisions to get cosmetic surgery. The discourses about cosmetic surgery that we find in public culture work variously to bolster its reputation, exploit its patients as spectacles, submit its patients to the psychiatric gaze, and challenge its politics.

Although many of these accounts offer insights that are useful and provocative, I want to critically reconsider them. In contrast to the assumptions underlying many of these approaches, my framework in this book does not begin with the idea that body practices bring out who we really are, and that the key to figuring out the meanings of cosmetic surgery lie only, or even primarily, in understanding the moral characters, mental health, or political consciousness of individual selves who undergo it. Following the insights of postmodern and poststructural social theory, I hold a skeptical view of attempts to declare the truth of individual subjectivities. This is in part because the meanings of neither our bodies nor our selves are as fixed as we often assume them to be. Moreover, social forces are interested in declaring the meanings of our bodies and selves for us. Some of them urge us to transform, improve, update, or change ourselves. Others urge us to embrace our authentic selves. Some do both. Our personal and social lives are full of tensions between stable and unstable conceptions of ourselves, our identities, and our bodies. My personal experience with cosmetic surgery underscored these tensions: I saw firsthand how in cosmetic surgery the body becomes a zone of social conflict, coded on the one hand as a sign of interior wellness and self-enhancement and on the other hand as a sign of moral, political, or mental weakness.

Within this conflict, women who get cosmetic surgery, as Kathy Davis found, use "discursive strategies" to make their decisions to have cosmetic surgery more understandable or defensible.[7] In other words, the narratives women tell to others—and perhaps even to themselves—about their own cosmetic surgeries are partly responses to how others define cosmetic surgery's meanings. For this reason, this book critically explores the discourses surrounding cosmetic surgery rather than critically exploring the cosmetic surgery patient herself. While Davis's account extensively researched what women say about their own decisions to have cosmetic surgery, my research examines what others—institutions, cultural and political interests, writers and scholars, doctors and lawyers—say about cosmetic surgery patients. It is their discourses that I want to interpret and deconstruct. The processes of producing the cosmetic surgery subject, or subjectivation, are the primary target of my thinking here. I believe this approach also tells us, indirectly, something important about the lived experience of getting cosmetic surgery.

The Normative Boundaries of Cosmetic Surgery

In chapter 1, "Visible Pathology and Cosmetic Wellness," I think about the relations between the body and the self, and I suggest how these relations are currently managed in the cultural production and definition of surgical bodies. In a number of ways, the body of cosmetic surgery is read as a code that reveals the pathology of the inner self. At the same time, in consumer culture we see the body's transformation as a sign of personal wellness and identity, a role exploited in cosmetic surgery discourse. I use poststructuralist theory, beginning with the work of Michel Foucault, as a framework for thinking about this contradiction. I argue for a theoretical approach that high-lights the ways in which cosmetic surgery culture produces a "hermeneutics of the self."

In chapter 2, "Normal Extremes: Cosmetic Surgery Television," I examine the commercialization of cosmetic surgery in contemporary popular culture. In particular, I look at the show *Extreme Makeover*. *EM* represents a celebratory attitude toward "extreme" cosmetic surgery. I describe how the show presents its own construction of "extreme" surgery as normal, expressing conventional ideas of the body and self and positioning cosmetic surgery as a tool for personal wellness and self-enhancement. I also address how the American Society for Plastic Surgeons officially responded to *Extreme Makeover*, in effect attempting to influence the social reception of cosmetic surgery television. The complicity and simultaneous ambivalence of cosmetic surgeons regarding *Extreme Makeover* and other shows reflect cosmetic surgery's awkward position as the most commercialized field of medicine.

Whereas *Extreme Makeover* presents the possibility of whole-body surgical overhauls without a trace of addiction or pathology, many feminists have had difficulty imagining any cosmetic surgery, however major or minor, that is not both pathological and addictive. In chapter 3, "Miss World, Ms. Ugly: Feminist Debates," I look at feminist depictions of cosmetic surgery. Many feminist critics of cosmetic surgery have described women's decisions to have cosmetic surgery as instances of internalized oppression that raise the risk of surgery addiction. Alternative accounts in feminist scholarship, to varying degrees, defend women's choices to get cosmetic surgery as rational expressions of women's agency. I suggest that these accounts not only correct some of the problems of feminist research on cosmetic surgery, but also imply the need to move beyond the "structure-agency" debate. I argue that feminism needs to be more critical of its own problematizations of cosmetic surgery, and suggest that the "structure-agency" debate is epistemologically and politically inadequate.

While a feminist reading blames patriarchal and consumer culture for the problems of cosmetic surgery, a psychiatric one focuses on individual pathology.[8] I pursue the meaning of pathological uses of cosmetic surgery in chapter 4, "The Medicalization of Surgery Addiction." Even though for the past two centuries cosmetic surgery was justified with psychological theories about self-esteem and inner well-being, it has also been read as a sign of mental ill-health. I describe how Body Dysmorphic Disorder, as the current primary diagnosis for cosmetic surgery addiction or obsession, operates as a medically constructed boundary for cosmetic surgery culture. This boundary is not fixed but rather in flux, and is negotiated, maintained, and reshaped by surgeons, psychotherapists, and the media, among others. I argue that current uses of BDD may place the burden of cosmetic surgery's problems unfairly on the shoulders of individual patients.

In chapter 5, "The Surgery Junkie as Legal Subject," I take up the legal construction of BDD in a court case called *Lynn G. v Hugo*. In *Lynn G.*, a middle-aged woman who saw her cosmetic surgeon over fifty times for various procedures decided to sue him for malpractice. The suit argued that her surgeon ought to have known that she had a body image disorder that made her obsessed with cosmetic surgery. The primary question of whether or not the doctor should have operated is never answered in the case. But the case introduces the surgery addict into the courtroom, and raises a whole range of questions about how doctors and patients can deal with extreme cases of cosmetic surgery. I describe the multiple interpretations of the addicted cosmetic surgery patient that appear in the case, which establishes the patient's psyche as the site of cosmetic surgery's troubles.

In chapter 6, "The Self and the Limits of Interiority," I argue that the ways we think about cosmetic surgery's ethical problems are dominated by the search for the truth of the subject of cosmetic surgery. I see this search as an example of the kind of "hermeneutics of the self" that Foucault claimed dominates modern society. I argue that a critical attitude toward this hermeneutics is essential for thinking about cosmetic surgery's power relations. I argue that in order to respond critically to cosmetic surgery, we must decenter the subject of cosmetic surgery, without losing grasp of how central she is to its power relations. I offer my own story of having cosmetic surgery in order to explore how we might approach the self of cosmetic surgery under these difficult epistemological circumstances.

Notes on Methodology

My arguments in this book are driven by theoretical concerns raised in contemporary philosophy, feminism, and social theory. I also rely on qualitative, interpretive research methods—primarily content analysis of popular, medical, legal, and specialty texts, and also interviewing. This is a mixed-methods approach, which I see as one of this book's particular strengths. At the same time, it also ensures that I will not have wholly covered, let alone exhausted, any one of these methods. There are many important issues in cosmetic surgery that I do not address at length. For instance, although I address a few aspects of racialization in cosmetic surgery, I do not thoroughly theorize or research this issue, even though I see racialization not only as one of cosmetic surgery's primary historical issues but also as one of its most pressing contemporary concerns. Further, I emphasize female cosmetic surgery patients over male, even though I discuss male patients as well. Women have historically made up the vast majority of cosmetic surgery patients, and female cosmetic surgery patients are most vulnerable to pathologization as well as political critique. Yet the phenomenon of male cosmetic surgery (which is on the rise) represents an important challenge to received understandings of cosmetic surgery. The work I present here, then, should not be read as an attempt to produce a fixed, inarguable truth about cosmetic surgery, or as a complete picture of its problems and issues. Instead, I offer an interpretive account that aims to illuminate some of the multiple and competing meanings about it that are emerging across disciplines and fields in academia, popular culture, medicine, psychiatry, and, to a limited extent, law.

Throughout the book I have used content analysis of textual material. Taking instruction from Deborah Sullivan's work *Cosmetic Surgery: The Cutting Edge of Commercial Medicine in America*, I examined how cosmetic surgeons and their professional organizations are framing cosmetic surgery through their press releases and newspaper interviews. Because of the dramatic recent changes in the cosmetic surgery landscape, and because I wished to build upon the work Sullivan has already done (which covered cosmetic surgery's history through the late 1990s), I limited my focus to the past ten years, and primarily looked at the past five years (2000–2005). I analyzed the press releases from the American Society of Plastic Surgeons and the American Society of Aesthetic Plastic Surgery between 2000 and 2005 to understand surgeons' official participation in managing media messages about cosmetic surgery, cosmetic surgery television, and BDD. I used content analysis to look at newspaper reporting on cosmetic surgery and BDD in twelve major newspapers (primarily from 1995 to 2005) to examine how BDD has been framed in the public discourse as a social problem. I also looked at the Web sites of surgery societies and individual surgeons and advertisements for cosmetic surgery published in various print and electronic media.

For my analysis of *Extreme Makeover* in chapter 2, I watched television shows on cosmetic surgery (particularly the pilot and first three seasons of *Extreme Makeover*), treating them as texts in the cultural studies tradition. For chapter 5, I examined court opinions from the New York State Supreme Court, Appellate Court, and Court of Appeals in the case *Lynn G. v Hugo*. I also looked at the psychiatric literature on Body Dysmorphic Disorder and the feminist literature on cosmetic surgery, treating both as discourses worth viewing comparatively. I describe my own viewing of Eve Ensler's performance of the surgery junkie in her play *The Good Body*. For my discussion of "cosmetic wellness" in chapter 1, I examined a number of popular books and Web sites on cosmetic surgery.

For chapters 2 and 4, I conducted twenty in-depth interviews with patients and doctors. I first conducted interviews with a small group of eight cosmetic surgery patients (all women), whom I found through a snowball method, which from a social scientific perspective is a nonprobability sample. Such a method is not generalizable, but it is useful because it helps a researcher observe shared cultural codes among people who are connected by some activity, behavior, or identification. As in studies by Kathy Davis, Debra Gimlin, and others, these interviews revealed the great extent to which women wrestled both with cultural encouragement to get cosmetic surgery and with significant social disapproval of such a decision. Like Gimlin, I suspected that women who get cosmetic surgery were strategic in describing their decisions to get surgery precisely because they expected moralistic or pathologizing treatment from others. I include some of the material from these interviews in this book, but I soon refocused my attention on the social contests that surround the moral, political, medical, and ethical meanings of getting cosmetic surgery. This includes a theoretically rich discussion, in chapter 3, of other, much more extensive interview studies, particularly those coming out of feminist research perspectives, which have struggled to make sense of women's narratives about their own cosmetic surgeries.

The other interviews I conducted were with doctors and other health-care workers whose geographic range spans the East and West Coasts of the United States. I again used a snowball method of finding participants. The doctors are in a variety of subspecialties in medicine (dermatology, ophthalmology, otolaryngology, psychiatry, and plastic surgery) and are all involved with cosmetic surgery in some respect. They are white men, except for two white female surgeons. The other health care workers were two women who had ancillary roles in cosmetic surgery offices. My interviews focused primarily on how cosmetic surgeons account for the recent surge in cosmetic surgery's popularity, and how they view their own patient populations in light of this.

There is also my autoethnographic account of own cosmetic surgery. In chapter 6 I describe my decision, in the midst of writing this book, to have cosmetic surgery. This involved consultations with five plastic surgeons, the surgery itself, and the pre-op and post-op visits, as well as the bodily, social, and familial experience of the surgery process. Without a doubt, having surgery gave me a different angle on the experience than I had from researching texts, speaking to doctors, and listening to other people's experiences. Although the physical aspects of the surgeries were challenging, interpersonal aspects of cosmetic surgery were even more difficult. Like Davis's interviewees, I received an "endless battery" of moral, political, and medical questions and interrogations by colleagues, friends, and acquaintances, while receiving encouragement from doctors (and, of course, advertisements and television programs).[9] At my first look from the vantage point of the patient, cosmetic surgery culture appeared to be almost simplistically bifurcated between opposing sides. Yet, as I hope to show here, there is a common focus to feminist, medical, psychiatric, and consumerist views: all of them point to the interrogation of the individual subject. Cosmetic surgery positioned me right in the midst of that interrogation, and in the last chapter I try to critically examine this experience.

1

Visible Pathology and Cosmetic Wellness

Cosmetic surgery transforms the outer, physical body, and this very fact renders it controversial. But I want to argue that the cultural, medical, and political relations of cosmetic surgery reach a great deal further than the physical, to what we think of as the self's interior, to the identity and psyche of the subject. In this chapter, I outline a range of treatments of cosmetic surgery, emerging from psychiatry, feminism, cosmetic medicine, and television, which are explored in this book. My project is to examine the ways in which they discursively establish the subjects of cosmetic surgery. Drawing from insights in contemporary social theory, I describe cosmetic surgery not only as a technology of body modification but also as a technology of psychic inscription. Cosmetic surgery instigates practices and discourses that define the self as well as the body, the personal interiority of the subject as well as its high-tech physique.

Visible Pathology

Cosmetic surgery is historically seen as a corruption of the natural body-self relation. The body that has undergone cosmetic surgery has been criticized for creating an untruthful representation of the inner self, for allowing an impression of the self that passes as someone else. This was one of the moral objections to cosmetic surgery reigning in the nineteenth and early twentieth centuries—that it was highly unnatural not just because it involved physical transformation but because it corrupted the normal, and even biologically driven, coding of a person's character on the body. Historian Sander Gilman describes how cosmetic surgery was feared for helping marginalized people pass into dominant groups, particularly with respect to race and criminality. "One great social fear in early twentieth century Europe and the United States," he writes, "was that the criminal, especially the Jew or black as criminal, would alter his appearance through the agency of the aesthetic surgeon and vanish into the crowd."[1] Such fear, of course, is highly essentialist, assuming that a person's essence is fixed by race, ethnicity, or some other category.

This essentialist logic still endures. We have seen it, for instance, in the relentless social fascination with Michael Jackson's cosmetic surgeries. With his increasingly pale skin and thinning nose, Jackson is variously seen as post-Black, as a denier of his racial heritage, and—combined with his gender- and age-defying body modifications—as a freak. Jackson's cosmetic alterations have become heightened to such spectacle that it has been difficult for us to avert our collective gaze. This is partly because he is seen as using technology to mask what we take to be his more authentic, biologically determined self, which would be Black, male, and middle-aged. In the late twentieth and twenty-first centuries, our collective unease may be informed not only by traditional attitudes about race transgression but also by a more modern public consciousness about the psychological effects of racism. As Kathy Davis puts it, "Ethnic cosmetic surgery evokes ambivalence. As a kind of surgical passing, it can be viewed as a symptom of 'internalized racism' or as a traitorous complicity with oppressive norms of appearance."[2]

Both historical and contemporary arguments against cosmetic surgery have generally assumed that the given body is authentic and the altered body is unnatural. But although the surgically transformed body has been seen as both immoral and politically incorrect, it is now also interpreted as pathological. Pathologizing discourses interpret the body of cosmetic surgery as a record of symptoms of psychological disorder. Jackson has been understood this way: as cultural studies scholar Nikki Sullivan describes, his surgeries have been repeatedly analyzed in the media, where his face is decoded by a range of experts. Jackson's modified face is, as Sullivan puts it, "read not only as the effect of an abusive childhood, but also as evidence of escalating psychological problems."[3] By repeatedly displaying images of his increasingly modified face as a visual illustration of his psychological biography, the media positions his physical transformation as indicative of increasing internal disorder. His modified face is interpreted as a code of his inner self that can be read easily by experts, if not by the public at large. While his seemingly weird tastes and unorthodox attitudes and actions are also pathologized, the surface body is—tautologically—offered as the material evidence for pathology, which includes, at the very least, cosmetic surgery addiction.[4]

Anomalous, spectacular bodies are easy targets for pathologization, but psychiatrists are now suggesting that all people who get cosmetic surgeries should be screened for mental pathology, particularly Body Dysmorphic Disorder. Body Dysmorphic Disorder is a diagnosis that is now being used to understand extreme cases of cosmetic surgery, especially what appears to be cosmetic surgery addiction, as well as to establish medical standards for patients' psychological attitudes toward their bodies. Despite its fairly short history as an official psychiatric disorder, BDD is a clinical buzzword in the current cosmetic surgery climate. The diagnosis of Body Dysmorphic Disorder is becoming much more widely understood as linked to cosmetic surgery, and in the public sphere, BDD is becoming a primary focus of cosmetic surgery's social problematization.

BDD is a category that defines the cosmetic surgery patient as pathological, or not, according to its diagnostic criteria. What interests me about the way BDD now circulates in the new cosmetic surgery climate is, to start, this very attempt to find the deep meanings of cosmetic surgery by identifying the pathologies of cosmetic surgery's subject, the (usually female) cosmetic surgery patient. I want to question the way BDD is being linked to cosmetic surgery. As I see it, the recent social problematization of BDD locates cosmetic surgery's troubles in the psyches of individual patients, and thus is a highly conservative response to controversial aspects of cosmetic surgery. Further, I argue that while some psychiatrists, journalists, and others fear that prime psychic features of cosmetic surgery patients can be defined by this new diagnosis, I think it is possible to suggest the reverse: that the increasing prominence of this diagnosis can shape the subjective meanings of cosmetic surgery. Social awareness of BDD plays an increasingly important role in our reception of cosmetic surgery, influences the ways in which we interpret the subjects of cosmetic surgery, and changes the social and intersubjective context in which people actually undergo surgery.

Psychiatry is not the only framework identifying the truth of cosmetic surgery patients. Feminism shares with psychiatry an interest in locating the subject of cosmetic surgery, in identifying the problematic psychic drive for surgical transformation. Although there are significant differences between feminist and psychiatric views on cosmetic surgery, the former generally square with the latter on at least two points: first, that cosmetic surgery reveals something deep about the individual self; and second, that what it reveals is pathological. Despite their objection to psychiatry's biologism and its apolitical stance, some feminists have applied the psychiatric language of self-mutilation and addiction to women who choose cosmetic surgery. They have described female cosmetic surgery patients as sick women whose psyches have been rendered pathological by patriarchy. But rather than look to biological or psychodevelopmental origins for this pathology, feminist treatments of cosmetic surgery, most of which come under the rubric of the "beauty ideals" perspective, see women's desires for cosmetic surgery as an outcome of beauty culture. This perspective indicts cosmetic surgery itself as politically problematic because of its reinforcement of beauty ideals, while perceiving women who use cosmetic surgery as victims of internalized oppression or false consciousness. Although some feminists, like Kathy Davis, defend women against charges of being dupes of patriarchy and emphasize women's agency as well as the structural relations of patriarchy, most feminist critiques of the practice, including Davis's, suggest that women who get cosmetic surgery suffer from bodily self-hatred as an effect of the pressures of patriarchal culture.

Feminism has offered the most powerful social critique

of cosmetic surgery thus far because it has insisted upon locating cosmetic surgery's problems not only in the psyches of individual patients but also in the industry itself. If cosmetic surgery is inherently suspect, immoral, or otherwise wrong, which is regularly assumed in both psychiatry and feminism, then we must be suspicious of the motives of cosmetic surgeons as well as patients, of the makers of breast implants as well as of the women who use them. In this sense, I find the history of feminist critiques of cosmetic surgery to be much less conservative, and ultimately more fairminded, than that of psychiatry. Yet I want to argue that feminism's own interest in establishing the truth of the cosmetic surgery patient has not been unproblematic.

I take up a more sustained critique of both feminist and psychiatric treatments of cosmetic surgery in later chapters. But for the moment, I want to argue that they both position cosmetic surgery as a visible pathology—they imagine that the psychic pathology of the cosmetic surgery patient is visibly expressed on the surface, on her or his body. Although no responsible psychiatrist or psychologist would literally diagnose a person by looking at her, I mean to suggest that these perspectives metaphorically treat the body as psychically inscribed. A number of assumptions inform this scenario. Most obvious is the sentiment against elective beautification surgery as self-harming, unnatural, or inauthentic, an idea based on assumptions about the natural, proper, healthy body as pristine or unmodified. But even more significant, I think, is that the self appears to be more or less fixed: there is a truth to the self that is expressed on the body, such as a medically pathological self or a politically corrupted or oppressed self. Similarly, cosmetic surgery is primarily defined by the interiority of the subject. This is especially so in psychiatric and psychological interpretations, but even feminists are open to this charge. Although feminists have been keen to examine the broader cultural contexts of cosmetic surgery, feminist approaches have been dominated by the agency-structure debate, which wrestles with the question of whether the politically oppressed self can be seen to make choices. Kathy Davis's work, which sees more possibility for agency in cosmetic surgery than do many other feminist interpretations, has opened up opportunities for feminist scholarship to complicate current understandings of cosmetic surgery.[5] Without the ability to believe that female cosmetic surgery patients can be normal rather than pathological, it is difficult to begin looking beyond the individual subject in our consideration of cosmetic surgery. If the cosmetic surgery patient is acting out of deep oppression and self-loathing—in other words, if she is in some way mentally ill—then it seems pointless to critique anything but her subjectivity. To move beyond Davis's contribution, in my view, feminism has to expand its focus far beyond the agency or oppression of the self as the primary site of cosmetic surgery's meanings.

There are other ways of thinking about cosmetic surgery and the relationship between the body and the self that it implies. We can think that the psychic self, as much as the body, can be inscribed. We can apply the insights of poststructural feminist Elizabeth Grosz, who argues that the body can be thought of as actively shaping the psyche as much as being shaped by it. Grosz describes her approach as "a kind of turning inside out and outside in of the body."[6] She uses the metaphor of the Möbius strip to explain this view of the body-self: each feeds into the other and it is impossible to separate them, or identify a discrete originality to either the outer body or the inner psyche. For Grosz, "people's experience of interiority is produced though the surface of the body, which we experience as already inscribed by cultural and social meanings of our bodies existing in social and cultural spaces."[7] In this view, neither psychic self nor physical body are fixed or natural or authentic, but rather continually created or in process. This post-essentialist perspective on the body and self means that we must think of the meanings of bodily practices such as cosmetic surgery as neither strictly internal nor external, but rather as intersubjective. Cosmetic surgery cannot be understood solely, then, through diagnosing the health or sickness, the authenticity or oppression, of the self.

One of the implications of a post-essentialist view, from the perspective of poststructural theory, is that discourses such as psychiatry that identify apparently fixed meanings for the self have to be critically examined, as Michel Foucault has written. Foucault famously argued that in modernity the soul became the prison of the body, as he wrote in *Discipline and Punish: The Birth of the Prison*.[8] What he meant was that the soul, or the authentic, true meaning of the inner self, has been invented, and that the body is the site for inscribing this truth. In his examples, the sexual self, the criminal self, the medically pathological self, and the insane self were each defined by modern institutions—sexology and education, criminology, medicine, and psychiatry. These definitions were normative, in the sense that they were created and enacted by institutional power and imposed on individual, embodied selves. He described how these disciplinary institutions offered the body up to new forms of knowledge. In the clinic, for example, the body was offered up to the new medical gaze.[9] In sexology, its sexuality was categorized according to new definitions of perversion.[10] In the school, the factory, the asylum, and the prison, the body was trained to be docile, and the individual was trained to self-police.

From Foucault's perspective, we can see medicine and psychiatry as practices of social control that produce certain kinds of bodies and psyches. Individual identities are shaped through the imposition of normative labels and categories, and bodies are made docile as they are socialized. In this sense, we can see cosmetic surgery as a disciplinary practice that medicalizes norms of beauty. Kathryn Pauly Morgan, synthesizing a beauty ideals perspective with a Foucaultian analysis, has argued that cosmetic surgery disciplines the body into and with beauty culture, creating docile bodies for cultural inscription that are underwritten with patriarchal and consumerist values.[11] But a Foucaultian perspective does not permit us to ignore other ways in which the body-subject is disciplined. Psychiatric understandings about Body Dysmorphic Disorder also operate in disciplinary ways, defining what constitutes a healthy attitude about the body through identifying unhealthy or pathological ones. I see many feminist arguments as similarly implicated.

Foucault's analysis pushes us far beyond the questions of whether or not cosmetic surgery is good or bad, and whether cosmetic surgery patients are healthy or sick. Foucault means for us to question the very epistemological basis of these questions. As Gilles Deleuze points out in his reading of Foucault, knowledge-power works through the dual mechanisms of visibility and articulability.[12] Visibility is the matter of what is seeable and why we see it and not something else. A field of visibility outlines the seeable, and what becomes self-evident, in a given era. For our purposes here, we might say that what is visible on the body, such as identity, pathology, health, wellness, or character, is historically shaped, linked to larger social formations and forces. We might ask, then, how do forces like consumer capitalism, the rise of individualism, current conceptions of health and illness, new configurations of medicine and technology, and other developments influence what we see when we look at the body? And then, what is not only see-able, but also sayable, about these things? What is speakable about the body, about identity, the self? What statements can be made? As Foucault showed in his historicizing treatments of social science, medicine, sexology, and psychiatry, fields of articulability are outlined by systems of knowledge. They are determining; they order the visible, have primacy over them. Visibilities are not created by discourse, but they are inseparable from discursive conditions "which open them up."[13]

Following this reading of Foucault, I see the bodies of cosmetic surgery as sites of visibility where the self is exposed. That we speak so much about the self and see it on the body's surface are not because we have found the real truth of cosmetic surgery, but because we are moved to consider and find this truth in historically specific ways. But I want to point out that in postmodern culture, the selves we see are in at least one sense actually far from fixed. They are not only pathological but also well. They are self-destructive, but also identity affirming. They are in touch with themselves and out of touch, inauthentic and authentic, extreme and normal. Thus the psychic and bodily inscriptions that Grosz identifies as co-constituted are not univocal and singular, but multiple and contradictory.

Cosmetic Wellness

If pathology is visible in cosmetic surgery, so is normalcy. The cosmetic surgery industry is now promoting "cosmetic wellness," whereby the tending and improvement of the outer body is coded as signifying a healthy inner self. This is a discursive strategy with historical precedent:

since the nineteenth century, surgeons argued that their practices improved patients' mental well-being by removing the burdens of abnormal appearance, which included racially or ethnically marked features.[14] Later, cosmetic surgeons appropriated the insights of Austrian psychologist Alfred Adler, who identified the so-called inferiority complex, to explain the benefits of cosmetic improvements. But current promotions of cosmetic wellness, which can be seen in cosmetic surgeons' advertisements, in their public relations campaigns, in their writings, and in the ways they talk about cosmetic surgery to the media and others, emphasize not only the amelioration of stigma but also improvement in overall body image and self-esteem as well as physical health and lifestyle.[15] Cosmetic wellness defines cosmetic surgery as a self-care practice that lays "the groundwork for greater all-around health and well-being, as well as an enhanced ability to take control of one's life," as Dr. Michelle Copeland, a Harvard-trained plastic surgeon from Manhattan, put it.[16] As Copeland told me in an interview, "How we look and how we feel are intimately related. If we look in the mirror and we look tired, we feel tired. If we look in the mirror and we look good, we feel good. If people say we look well, we feel well."[17] This might be a clichéd understanding of the body and self, but cosmetic surgeons mean it literally. According to Copeland, a person with a good self-image who cares about her well-being will not only get liposuction or a face lift when she needs it, however this is determined, but will also stay fit, eat well, exercise, and live life to the fullest.

Copeland wrote her own book extolling the virtues of cosmetic wellness; other doctors have articulated this perspective through the news and entertainment media. In her analysis of articles on cosmetic surgery in women's magazines, sociologist Abigail Brooks describes how cosmetic doctors and journalists discursively link cosmetic surgery with health and wellness. She describes how technologies are equated with "workouts" for one's face and body, with getting one's skin and body "into shape," and as part of a healthy lifestyle. For example, "as an article in *Vogue* magazine explains, people who have been working out for a year but still 'cannot lose the fat' make 'ideal candidates' for microlipo. According to Dr. Bellin: 'The solution is modest lipo, true body sculpting used as an add-on to a healthy lifestyle.'"[18] This logic surfaces not just in *Vogue* magazine; it is also championed by the American Society for Aesthetic Plastic Surgery (ASAPS), which funded a survey-based study on the psychological makeup of facelift patients. Its findings: while facelift patients may be significantly more dissatisfied with their appearance than what they called the "typical American," they are also significantly more invested in not only appearance but also fitness and health.[19] Thus, cosmetic surgery can reflect one's whole psychosocial identity as healthy and self-attentive.[20] The cosmetic surgery profession also argues that lifestyle is improved with cosmetic wellness. For example, as another professional society, the American Society of Plastic Surgeons (ASPS) describes, a tummy tuck can help a person have a "less restrictive lifestyle": "Imagine feeling inhibited in your daily activities because you're extremely self-conscious about a certain area of your body . . . prospective tummy tuck (abdominoplasty) patients have great dissatisfaction with the appearance of their abdomens, which ultimately affects how they feel and act in certain situations."[21] Further, cosmetic surgeons argue, in direct contrast to feminist critiques, that a cosmetic surgery patient might even treat depression or a problem with her body image surgically. In fact, the very "purpose of cosmetic surgery," says Dr. Gregory Borah, on behalf of the ASAPS, "is to improve a person's psychological functioning by modifying their body image."[22]

Cosmetic wellness represents not only what feminists have critiqued as the medicalization of beauty but also a much broader shift toward lifestyle medicine. In postmodern culture we have seen a transition from a biomedical culture to what is often called a "biopsychosocial" one, which enlarges our interest in health to increasingly include its social and psychic aspects. Beyond this, though, the focus on health has dramatically expanded to include maintenance, lifestyle, and appearance, while transforming the patient into a consumer. As consumers, we scout the Web for the latest health research, preventative measures, medical trials, and cosmetic procedures. We assume greater responsibilities in our exchanges with doctors and clinics. We take on a wider array of body projects related to health, from dieting to yoga. We take more elective medicines, from those to improve our sex lives to those that limit menstruation, or help us sleep, concentrate, relax, perform athletically, or look better. In all, the trend toward lifestyle medicine has "massively expanded" the subjects of health care from sick bodies to the whole population.[23] Gilles Deleuze accounts for this by describing how disciplinary society has given way to what he calls "control society," which includes "the new medicine 'without doctor or patient' that singles out potential sick people and subjects at risk."[24] Whereas the sick body was once the primary territory of medicine, appearance and beauty are now increasingly seen as occasions for medical consumerism, and healthy bodies are regularly tuned up both inside and out. Cosmetic surgery is the archetypical form of this kind of medicine. It utilizes a vastly expanded role for medicine, positions the patient as a consumer who pursues medical resources for lifestyle maintenance, appeals to healthy people, and links appearance and beauty with physical and mental fitness.

The rhetoric of cosmetic wellness, combined with increasing public concern over cosmetic surgery's pathological subjects, have set the stage for new discussions of what constitutes the good patient, the good psyche, and the good body image in cosmetic surgery. For instance, the American Society for Aesthetic Plastic Surgery, in the wake of public debate over BDD, has established an outline of how much cosmetic surgery a person should get. "How much cosmetic surgery is too much?" asks the ASAPS. The answer is that it "depends on the reasons it is chosen, when it is chosen, and the patient's expectations. A patient who has a strong personal desire for self-improvement and is able to identify specific, realistic goals for surgery is likely to be a suitable candidate for one or more procedures."[25] Lest we be uncertain about what those goals should be, the ASAPS published a timeline that identifies what women's concerns might be at which age, and which cosmetic surgeries address them. Not surprisingly, it is a pretty expansive list, establishing a regimen over one's adult lifetime that, if one took the advice to its maximum, would amount to approximately fifteen surgical procedures, along with numerous laser treatments and dozens of injections, sustained over a span of forty to fifty years.[26] The promotion of a healthy regimen of cosmetic surgery over one's adult lifetime, in contrast to cosmetic surgery addiction, depends upon outlining a proper body image and body-self relationship. If the surgeries are undertaken in the right order, with the right mental framework, and with the right beauty concerns, cosmetic surgery can come to be seen like regularly scheduled body maintenance.

What distinguishes cosmetic surgery addiction from cosmetic wellness is not the number of surgeries, then, but rather the interior self, the psychic character of the subject. Correspondingly, there is now a deluge of self-help information in popular culture on the psychology of cosmetic surgery. One example is psychologist Joyce Nash's self-help book on cosmetic surgery, where she asks readers to take a quiz called "Are You a Good Candidate for Cosmetic Surgery?"[27] In a series of questions, she asks readers to account for their interest in cosmetic surgery, to identify what instigated the interest, and to assess their expectations for surgery. The lessons of the quiz are, in my reading, as follows: cosmetic surgery does not substantially improve one's romantic life or employment situation; cosmetic surgery that is designed to please someone else is a bad idea; life crises are bad times for cosmetic surgery, and impulsive decisions are bad; there is pain and physical trauma to cosmetic surgery, and thinking otherwise is bad; needing "a lot of comfort and tender loving care from a doctor or special attention from the doctor's staff" is not good.[28] In contrast, good candidates for surgery: do it for themselves; carefully consider their options; are generally happy with themselves; and take cosmetic surgery seriously. Criteria like these are widely discussed in cosmetic surgery popular culture, although there is some disagreement among the various sources offering advice. The self-help authors Charlee Ganny and Susan Collini, for instance, argue that it is acceptable to want cosmetic surgery in order to get a better love life, or to compete in the job market.[29] And the ASAPS suggests that "Over an individual's lifetime, there may be various stages at which cosmetic surgical or nonsurgical enhancements can improve the quality of life," thus affirming that rather broad goal.[30] Although there is no undisputed norm that establishes the proper body image, the right attitude, and the correct aims for cosmetic surgery, rehearsing what these might or should be appears to be the goal of the pop-psychology and consumerist cosmetic surgery discourse.

Cosmetic surgery is now linked not only to psychological health but also other aspects of identity. As I describe in chapter 2, on what became the wildly popular television show *Extreme Makeover*, cosmetic surgery is said to help the body express its real self. In one case, a fat man who works as a personal trainer is returned to his true, formerly thin self with high-tech assistance. In the story *Extreme Makeover* tells, he becomes not less but more like the person he really is through surgical body modification. In another narrative, a woman reclaims the "sleeping beauty" inside of her; others reclaim their youthful selves, which are more authentic than the middle aged selves they now see in the mirror. As I argue, *Extreme Makeover* accomplishes the extreme transformation of the body through highly normalizing narratives linked to reigning ideas about the authenticity and primacy of individual identities. In its selling of cosmetic surgery, cosmetic medicine realigns inner and outer selves, establishing the proper relationship between surface appearance and interior identity.

This is nowhere more apparent than in the development of "ethnically appropriate" cosmetic surgery. On *Extreme Makeover*, a former Philipina beauty queen regains her looks with the help of cosmetic surgery. But for her facial surgery, *Extreme Makeover* made a point of pursuing "ethnically appropriate" cosmetic surgery, reflecting a trend in the industry toward the development of specialized knowledge about non-white patients. While the racialization of beauty has long been part of cosmetic surgery's history, now the promotion of ethnically appropriate surgery is informed by multiculturalism. Instead of aiming to erase racial difference, ethnically appropriate cosmetic surgery identifies differences in the needs and interests of racial and ethnic groups. Figuring out the variations among ethnic skin types in terms of likely reactions to surgery, lasers and other procedures are now seen as a quality-of-care matter among cosmetic surgeons.[31] But as the *Cosmetic Surgery Times* puts it, the "main caveats in these areas involve cultural features."[32] Such features include attitudes about eye shape among Asians, attitudes about noses among African Americans, Latinos' ideals of body shape, and so on. Ethnically targeted cosmetic surgery now aims to rethink Eurocentric beauty ideals in order to preserve the ethnic features of the person, and to honor her or his racial heritage.[33]

Such attempts may be welcome for some people of color who have been frustrated with the cosmetic surgery industry's homogenized view of beauty. But although ethnically appropriate cosmetic surgery might answer current bioethical criticisms about race and cosmetic surgery, it surely generates new ones. For instance, it reifies racial categories, universalizing beauty within ethnic groups and utilizing an essentialist logic that emphasizes innate rather than social meanings of race. It also demands that individuals see their authentic selves in racially or ethnically specific terms. As Kathy Davis points out, "patients who 'reject' their ethnic background [now] make poor candidates for cosmetic surgery."[34] To my mind, this insistence that individuals identify as properly Latino or Asian is not any more ethical than insisting that they look white. Such logic affirms a normative idea about the proper relationship between the body and the self, where the body's role is to articulate the self's real, authentic identity.

This logic positions cosmetic surgery as a practice of self-definition. In postmodern culture, the body has an expanded role in personal identity. Bodies are now interpreted as highly specific signifiers of individual identities. They are supposed to suggest, as philosopher Alphonso Lingus puts it, "the very expression, moment by moment, of an inward spirit, or a person belonging to himself."[35] To explain this view of the self as up for individual construction, social theorist Anthony Giddens has described how contemporary life is marked by a sense of uprootedness, mobility, and a loss of traditional anchors for our senses of self.[36] Thus, identity is now less proscribed than achieved. As Giddens sees it, we now have greater opportunities than ever before for self-expression and elective identity. It is now our task to create a personalized sense of who we are, and we do so by undertaking identity projects. These are often made up of consumer practices that increasingly take place in the arena of the body. As body theorist Chris Shilling puts it, affluent Westerners now see the body "as an entity which is in the process of becoming: a project which should be worked out and accomplished as part of an individual's self-identity."[37] Further, current uses of technology escalate the project beyond previously understood limits. As medical sociologist Bryan Turner has it, "the transformation of medical technology has made possible the construction of the human body as a personal project."[38] In *Extreme Makeover*'s rendering of this situation, cosmetic surgery not only helps us be the people we want to be, but might actually be necessary to represent who we really are.

But as I see it, the neoliberalism of Gidden's theory of the late modern self, the idea that society treats the body and self as opportunities for self-creation, does not give enough emphasis to the political economies underlying identity projects. My more poststructural view worries that our identity practices are influenced at least as much by structural forces as by individual agency or creativity.

Contemporary Western identities cannot be separated from consumer capitalism. As Deleuze points out, capitalism not only sells products and services but also codes meanings—for instance, the identities that we are supposed to be expressing when wear that sort of wardrobe, engage in this sort of lifestyle, or undergo that cosmetic surgery.[39] Further, not only is the symbolism of the body for sale but the very ability of the body to signify in such escalated ways is also a part of its commodification. While bodies have always been marked to express social meanings, consumer capitalism speeds up the body's morphing and its role in identity production. As Shilling points out, the very production of the self is now wrapped up in the continual transformation of the body. Postmodern capitalism orchestrates the construction of not only individual bodies but also inner selves—whether healthy selves, empowered selves, beautified selves, authentic selves, or selves in touch with ourselves—through the aggressively commercial targeting of intimate, personal body-self relationships.

Like the pathologies of cosmetic surgery, then, I see its healthful or normative expressions as socially produced. The normal self of the twenty-first century, who embraces certain attitudes about fitness and lifestyle, views medicine as a broad personal resource, envisions the body as a medium for individual narrative, and affirms her authentic identity, is not inherently proper and authentic but rather is a historical production. So is the depth of meaning that she is supposed to be expressing with her body.

Inner Selves and Social Meanings

Cosmetic surgery culture not only creates a surface appearance that is normatively ideal but also produces that appearance's psychic meanings. When Michael Jackson's face is read as a signifier of the true meaning of his inner self, it is decoded according to standards that are influenced by racialized, gendered norms of appearance. When he fails to look Black and middle-aged, he is understood as a surgery addict and a sick person. The timeline offered by the ASAPS suggests that we might want to undergo at least as many cosmetic surgeries as he, but we must avoid the enfreakment that his extreme surgical project seems to effect (as well as such obvious racial passing). A good candidate for cosmetic surgery will now have a specific set of attitudes about such surgery, will undertake it for the right reasons at the right time, and will want to honor her authentic inner self (even her ethnically appropriate self). A bad candidate for cosmetic surgery will have the wrong attitude and the wrong reasons, will want to change the wrong body parts at the wrong times, and will want to erase her ethnic or racial identity. Thus, as I see it, the dominant logics of contemporary cosmetic surgery now reach significantly beyond beauty ideals. Such logics depend upon essentialist notions of authentic inner selves. They require an understanding of the body and its surface as a signifier of authentic inner meaning. They recruit psychiatric strategies—or, alternatively, political or consumerist ones—to decode the meanings they find.

Is there another way to read cosmetic surgery? A postessentialist, poststructural view insists that there are no fixed, inherent meanings to the self, and further, that the body-self relationship is a historically specific production. The visibility of the body and self, or the body-as-self, is not inevitable, and its articulability is shaped by power relations. Thus, as Suzanne Fraser tells us in *Cosmetic Surgery, Gender, and Culture*, the subject of cosmetic surgery is a cultural product; she is produced through and within the discourses that define her, as well as through her own subjectivity.[40] Nikki Sullivan's argument about Michael Jackson anticipates this. She wants to find the meanings of Michael Jackson's body modifications not in his psyche, but elsewhere. In Sullivan's account of Michael Jackson, the significant meanings of his modified face do not derive simply from some inner essence of self that he is expressing: they are also outside of him. Sullivan implies that they are located in the transgression of racial and gender norms; in the discourses of psychiatry and psychology that use Jackson's body to generate knowledge about his psyche; in related feminist treatments of body modifiers as self-mutilators; and in the entertainment media, which present his body over and over again for spectacle. In other words, the significance of Michael Jackson's body lies not in the depth of his inner self, but in the relation between the depth and its surface, which we invest with what Deleuze would call "cultural intensity." Thus it is not of Michael Jackson whom we should try to make sense, but rather of what is visible and sayable about him.

As I suggest in this book, there are multiple ways in which we look to the intentions and psychosomatic history of the individual cosmetic surgery patient to find meaning. Some have searched for the deep psychic pathologies behind cosmetic surgery—its link to psychoanalytic problems, personal pathologies, and diagnosable psychiatric disorders. Highly commercial discourses about cosmetic surgery, like those found on television, read signs of interior health or statements of identity. Feminists have looked for signs of internalized political oppression and gendered self-hatred. Surgeons have made their own observations about cosmetic surgery patients, and have recently been asked to screen them, and to look for predictable, reliable ways to delineate good and bad patients. They have generated distinctions between good and bad reasons and right and proper time-lines for cosmetic surgery, and they have articulated the kind of body-self attitude that a patient ought to have.

But are cosmetic surgery's meaning and significance really found in the normalcy or pathology of the individual person? Feminists have always rejected the individualizing moves of psychiatry, but I want to suggest that a critical response to cosmetic surgery has to reach much further than feminist analyses of cosmetic surgery have done thus far. Following Grosz, I want to turn cosmetic surgery's meanings "inside out." I want to trace the discursive construction of cosmetic surgery subjects. Individual, personal, and psychic meanings of the body do, of course, exist alongside social meanings. But I would argue that our attempts to extract and decipher them reveal at least as much about our social norms and instruments of understanding as they do about individual truths. As Deleuze argues in his assessment of Foucault, "Truth is inseparable from the procedure establishing it."[41] And in cosmetic surgery discourse, there are multiple processes establishing multiple truths, which are sometimes allied with each other and sometimes in contradiction. I argue that in cosmetic surgery culture, these processes are at work coding the psyche as much as they are decoding the body.

In this chapter, I have attempted to outline a theoretical perspective that begins to shift the discussion away from debating the truth of the cosmetic surgery subject in order to consider the debates themselves as practices of subjectivation. My perspective asks for more thinking on not simply the problems but also on the problematizations of cosmetic surgery. In Deleuze's account of Foucault, he writes that: "We are not asking only about the objects with which we begin, the qualities we follow and the states of things in which we are located . . . but also how can we extract visibilities from these objects, qualities and things, how do these visibilities shimmer and gleam and under what light, and how does this light gather . . . ? Furthermore, what are the variable subject-positions of these visibilities? Who occupies and sees them?"[42] This shift from looking at the objects themselves to looking at the ways we look at, see, and articulate these objects is an epistemological challenge. In the next chapters, I trace just some of what gleams and shimmers on the bodies of cosmetic surgery patients. I point out what is visible, in Foucault's sense, as well as what is sayable or being said about them. I address who the subjects of cosmetic surgery turn out to be, as they appear on television, in surgeons' accounts, in feminist politics, in psychiatry and, in one case, in the courtroom. And ultimately, I make a case for the need to establish an alternative approach to thinking about cosmetic surgery that is not caught up in what Foucault calls a "hermeneutics of the self," obsessed with establishing the truth of the individual subject.

2

Normal Extremes

Cosmetic Surgery
Television

When three people in their twenties and thirties, Luke, Stephanie, and Stacey, collectively underwent over twenty-five hours of cosmetic surgery, documented in a two-hour special episode of network television, we were witnessing the beginning of a significant shift in the public discourse about cosmetic surgery. Before then, the idea that ordinary people would willingly expose their cosmetic surgeries, allowing millions of viewers to examine their "before" and "after" bodies in such detail, seemed unlikely. But more incredible was the very premise of popularizing an extreme surgical makeover, in which people would undergo not just one but numerous cosmetic surgeries to drastically change their appearance. This happened on the show *Extreme Makeover* (*EM*), which first aired on ABC on December 11, 2002. Since then, cosmetic surgery has become a regular staple of television fare, featured on other reality shows as well as many documentaries, dramas, and other programs.

Television is one socially important place where the meanings of cosmetic surgery are being generated. Henry

Giroux describes television shows as "popular pedagogies" because, for better or worse, they circulate not only information but also social meanings, norms, and values to their audiences.[1] And as Suzanne Fraser suggests, cosmetic surgery finds such "rich expression in the media" that it demands an analysis of its "impact on culture."[2] Although the idea of doing multiple or extreme cosmetic surgeries was not invented by television, I describe in the second half of this chapter how cosmetic surgeons see television as responsible for at least some of cosmetic surgery's recent market expansion, as well as for the public's understanding of what cosmetic surgery is, what it means, who should use it, and how much is acceptable. In this chapter, I describe *Extreme Makeover*'s vision of cosmetic surgery, and later explain cosmetic surgeons' simultaneous complicity and unease with its representations. *Extreme Makeover* generated what were promoted as extreme instances of bodily transformation while at the same time producing sympathetic, socially acceptable cosmetic surgery patients. Like some of the other celebrations of cosmetic surgery I described in chapter 1, the show promoted the body as a key to expressing and even establishing one's true identity, while identifying cosmetic surgery as a practice of self-expression, personal wellness, and self-care. At least rhetorically, it managed to create extreme surgery without casting its characters as surgery junkies. At the same time, this show and its successors are now part of the debates on cosmetic surgery excess.

Real Bodies on Reality Television

Extreme Makeover is part of the genre of reality television, the appeal of which is that its participants are not actors using scripts, but purportedly real people. Thus, the audience can empathize with the participants to a much greater degree than they can with actors. But as cultural studies scholar Amanda Klein points out, audiences are also well aware that reality television creates people that are essentially characters, in the sense that they are constructed—chosen, filmed, and edited through the high level of mediation of television production.[3] Reality television thus has a complicated relationship with its audiences; it asks them to relate to the people on the show as real, but aims to create situations, characters, and events that are more spectacular and entertaining than ordinary life. *EM's* version of extreme cosmetic surgery fulfills both tasks. However constructed the characters and situations may appear, the bodies undergo actual surgery by real surgeons.

Extreme Makeover was structured in the following way: cosmetic surgery makeovers would be granted as prizes to participants who had competed to win by writing applications, which were essentially stories about their desires for bodily improvement. *Extreme Makeover* would pay a team of experts—surgeons, dentists, dermatologists, and so on— to suggest and perform procedures, ranging from surgeries to teeth whitening and chemical peels. The participants would not only be given the rhinoplasty, tummy tuck, or breast lift they had especially wanted but they would also get a whole range of additional procedures that would beautify them. For six weeks, they would stay in hotels, hospitals, and clinics paid for by *EM*, isolated from friends and family. At the end of six weeks, each participant would be given a party, what the show called the "Big Reveal," where he or she would be reintroduced to their amazed friends, family, and loved ones in new haircuts, clothing, and makeup, but most important, in permanently, surgically changed bodies.

The cosmetic surgery projects of *Extreme Makeover* are

presented, by definition, as extreme. But what exactly is extreme about these makeovers? Whereas a makeover once implied changes in wardrobe, hair, and makeup, in every episode of the show, participants also undergo multiple cosmetic surgeries. Moreover, the cosmetic surgery of *EM* is astonishing in terms of its scale–multiple body parts, many hours of surgery, and only six weeks to transform its participants. The surgeons target noses and chins, cheeks and foreheads, eyes and lips, teeth, breasts, stomachs, thighs, and buttocks. They regularly use implants in the chin and breasts. They apply liposuction to faces, necks, and bodies. They undertake body lifts—in one case, a "triple body lift" that required three surgeons operating at once. They rearrange faces and redraw profiles. Dentists pull and cap teeth. Dermatologists resurface the skin. *Extreme Makeover* presents extreme cosmetic surgery as a set of practices that can radically change one's appearance, erase twenty years of aging, or transform ugly ducklings into swans. The show takes what it considers average or uglier than average people and gives them the looks of movie stars, and pays for tens of thousands of dollars worth of surgery, sums far beyond the reach of the participants and the vast majority of the audience. In these ways, as one family member observed on the show, "they aren't kidding when they say *extreme* makeover."

But the meanings of the extreme makeover reach far beyond the physical. Like other shows of its genre, *Extreme Makeover* uses not only a voice-over narrator but also what cultural studies scholar Hugh Curnutt calls "confessional-reflexivity," where participants' own views and insights "function as mechanisms that drive the program's narrative by embedding dialogue of a 'profound' nature throughout the text."[4] By using the voices of participants themselves (often in the intimate video-cinematic code of the close-up shot), such shows bring audiences emotionally closer to them. In fact, the subjective experiences of the participants are the show's true subject. Essential to *EM*'s presentation of cosmetic surgery is that participants would be able to show not just their bodies, but also their lives, as changed for the better if they were to be surgically altered. Applicants for *EM* are asked to answer the question, "If you were to receive 'The Extreme Makeover' in what ways would your life be altered?"[5] The participants' stories, told through interview clips (without an on-camera interviewer, as if they were confessing straight to the audience) as well as the voice-over narrator, emphasize the impact cosmetic surgery has on individuals' psychological health and definitions of self. Nearly every narrative explains participants' subjective experiences of surgical body transformation as life-altering.

Revealing the Inner Self

Luke

In the stories of *EM*, each participant is presented as both transformed and restored by cosmetic surgery. Luke gets cosmetic surgery in order to express his true inner self. He was a twenty-nine-year-old personal trainer who taught other people how to get fit, but he had been seriously obese himself. His story is about an "old" fat body at odds with its thinner self. We are told that Luke had found it humiliating that his body seemed to belie, in the words of the narrator, what he "stood for" in his career— personal fitness and self-discipline. By the time he applied to be on the show, he had already lost 125 pounds through diet and exercise. But instead of looking fabulous, Luke had been left with hanging skin around his abdomen that presumably would never go away, marring his good looks and constantly reminding him of his old, fatter self. The narrator of the show describes the sense of unfairness this created for him. He had worked hard to lose weight, but a thin, beautiful body eluded him nonetheless. As Luke himself told the camera, he was "trying to get rid of that [fat] person" for good when he applied to get an abdominoplasty on *Extreme Makeover*.

After we see Luke informed at home—ecstatic—that he won a makeover, we see him attending consultations with *EM*'s primary cosmetic surgeon, Dr. Garth Fisher, who will perform not only the abdominoplasty he desired but also a rhinoplasty to straighten and reduce the size of his nose. Dr. Fisher shows Luke a digitally altered image of his face on a computer screen before the surgery. He also describes the abdominoplasty procedure, saying, "we're going to make an incision across here, and then we're going to take this [handful of skin] and we're going to throw it away." We see Luke wearing a surgical gown, being pushed in a wheelchair, and lying on the operating table under anesthetic, connected to IV tubes. Under the hands of Dr. Fisher, along with an anesthesiologist and surgical nurse, we see graphic images of the surgery itself, including the knife cutting into skin. Later, Luke is in recovery, at times sitting in a wheelchair and other times lying in a hospital bed and being tended by a nurse. Initially he can't walk; later he uses a walker to get around. When he is fully recovered, he finishes his makeover with teeth whitening and hair implants. The procedures that *EM* provided made him feel "like a whole new person," as his mother put it in an interview at the Big Reveal, where the transformed Luke has stepped out to the applause of his family and friends.

Luke may feel like a new person, but creating a new self in these stories is really about allowing the real, true, or more proper self to be restored or revealed. Because the bodies are presented as highly pathological, the physical transformation is a process of restoration or repair, of bringing the body closer to its more authentic and proper self, as opposed to a process of experimentation, invention, or of creating something wholly new. In this logic, the real inner self of the patient is masked by the current physical body. In Luke's story, his proper body is thin rather than fat. Likewise, his real identity is not a fat or undisciplined self, but rather a fit and disciplined self. Through abdominoplasty, Luke's body-self relationship is realigned so that his body more properly identifies his true self. Thus, after his surgery, Luke's mother reassures us that he "still looks like Luke, only better." Tellingly, in this episode, the Big Reveal is also described as a "coming-out party."

Stephanie

The importance of transforming one's body in order to affirm a hidden or masked part of one's self is also expressed by the other participants. Before her makeover, Stephanie is presented as a homely, self-sacrificing single mother burdened with not only an ugly nose but also a life full of domestic tedium and financial strain. She is shown at home in the kitchen, carrying a laundry basket and performing other domestic tasks. She describes herself as a person who "could never have afforded a makeover like this." In any case, she tells us that she would have felt guilty spending money on herself, since she would have been "taking it from [her] own children." The makeover she will get addresses some significant problems with her psyche as well as her looks. Her rhinoplasty, we are told by the narrator, is going to fix a psychological complex she has had since the third grade, when her childhood friends teased her for having a "hook nose." Dr. Fisher even jokes with her about the ugliness of her nose, saying after the surgery:

"We got rid of that bump. We carried it off in a bucket." To make matters worse, we are told that during pregnancy, Stephanie's weight "ballooned out of control," and so she also needs liposuction. In addition, Stephanie will get breast implants and Lasik eye surgery, topped off with cosmetic dentistry and makeup and hairstyling.

As Stephanie undergoes over ten hours of surgery, we see graphic images of her body on the surgical table, including a shot of one of her breast implants being inserted. Afterwards, during recovery, she has bruising, swelling, and discomfort. But once the bandages are off, Stephanie announces that this is "the new me." Examining herself in the mirror, she exclaims, "I don't feel like I look like a mom anymore!" Of course, Stephanie isn't really abandoning her role as a mother, but she is delighted to abandon what she sees as the unglamorous body and face of a typical mom. After her whole face is surgically altered, she says that she has become "the person I always dreamt of." The person Stephanie always dreamt of being, it appears, is not the lonely single mother she has become, but neither is she a wholly new character, or a truly different self. Instead, this person is her inner, real, or better self that she might have become if her life circumstances had turned out differently. As in the marketing lingo of the Army that one can "be all you can be," what is suggested here is that one's hidden potential can be discovered and affirmed. You can look like your better self. You can embrace your existential possibilities that were stunted by an ugly body or a strained, difficult life.

Stacey

Stacey, too, has a better, truer self waiting to come out. Like Stephanie's bumpy nose and Luke's extra flesh, Stacey's face is abject. By her own account, her face has "no profile, no chin, fat cheeks, and a bird beak." Stacey, a health-care worker in her early thirties, is introduced as a single woman who has a hard time getting dates. Soon after we meet her, we are shown a photograph of Stacey in high school, where she played on the boys' football team. Alongside her male teammates, Stacey wears a typical uniform of protective shoulder pads, jersey, and helmet. Like the images of Luke at the gym and of Stephanie doing the laundry, this image is presented as an important clue to the meaning of Stacey's story. Perhaps the photograph is supposed to say what is too rude to say aloud: she looks more like a man than a woman, and thus has acted like one, too. As an adult, her homely looks have rendered her lonely and unconfident. In another scene, Stacey sits at a bar with her girlfriends, talking and laughing, but without any interested man in sight. In fact, the narrator tells us that it is Stacey's "heartfelt desire to attract the man of her dreams [which] makes her an ideal candidate for an extreme makeover." The rhinoplasty, chin implant, facial liposuction, and eyebrow lift that *EM*'s doctors prescribe are literally intended to rebuild her face, but are also intended to rebuild her prospects for love and happiness. After seeing herself digitally remade on a computer monitor in the surgeons' office, Stacey tells us this experience "gave me all kinds of hope" about the possibilities of technological transformation. Wearing a hospital gown in preparation for surgery, Stacey remarks that she is "really nervous, but excited to know that I'm starting my new life."

The new life that Stacey wants is a typical, heterosexually successful one: she needs the new looks to find a man. Happily, we are led to believe that she will get what she is looking for. After the makeover that reshapes her entire face, Stacey looks much more like the Hollywood ideal of female beauty. She enters the room at her Big Reveal to see her astonished family and friends crying and applauding, amazed at the transformation. Like all of the women at their Big Reveals, she wears the kind of gown, jewels, high heels, and hairstyle that one would expect from an actress at the Oscars. But in this episode, we also follow Stacey as she "reenters her life," the scene of which is a bar. The camera shows men looking at her approvingly as she walks by. As I read it, Stacey's is a heterosexual coming-out story: from cross-dressing football player to proper female beauty. Now men will see Stacey for the real woman she is, instead of the mannish, unfeminine person suggested by her old visage.

Tess

Extreme Makeover describes the potential of medical technology as limitless, but the surgeries don't explore just any possibility for transformation. Instead, the patients are presented as having ideal or more authentic versions of their selves that are hidden or obscured by the body's given materiality. Stacey is a woman and is supposed to look like one. Luke is self-disciplined and is supposed to be thinner. Stephanie's nose should never have been so bumpy, and her body should be as it was before pregnancy marred it. Moreover, Stephanie should simply look more glamorous, because despite her dreary, financially strapped life as a single mom, she's a real woman on the inside. For Tess, an Asian former beauty queen presented in the third season, such an ideal version of the body was once the foundation of her identity. Now aged forty-four and a mother of three, Tess is described as having a "ruined" body: "Multiple pregnancies and a large cesarean section scar ruined the body of this former beauty pageant queen. The Extreme Team now gives Tess the opportunity to regain the beauty that once accompanied her indestructible spirit."[6] Tess is restored to her former beauty-pageant self through abdominoplasty. Like many of the narratives about women on *EM*, Tess's story describes how motherhood and aging damage the bodies and distort the physical selves of women. Her damaged body exists in problematic contrast with her imperishable, fixed spirit.

But Tess's cosmetic surgery is complicated, the narrator tells us, by her ethnicity. Even though she was already considered beautiful, Tess is treated to a rhinoplasty along with her other procedures. The nose job will create a new and ostensibly improved look to her face. However, *EM* wants to ensure that the face she gets will be the right one, ethically speaking. Unlike most *EM* patients, 81 percent of whom are white, Tess is Philipina.[7] Tess is described as "accomplishing her makeover despite the concerns of ethnic plastic surgery," because for her face *EM* employed the services of a specialist in so-called ethnic cosmetic surgery.[8] Tess's doctor, Jon Perlman, is said to have expertise in performing surgery on ethnic minorities, and has studied ethnic variations in beauty and beauty ideals. Such an approach to ethnic cosmetic surgery patients is becoming more commonplace; ethnic cosmetic surgery is presented as more multicultural, less whitening, and thus more acceptable for people of color. But the message of ethnic cosmetic surgery is consistent with the overall goals of cosmetic surgery as presented on *EM*: to ensure that the true inner self is properly reflected in the physical body. In this story, while Tess will regain what she once had, she will also retain her ethnic authenticity. Her new and improved body will be exactly in line with her purportedly authentic self.

Normalcy, Self-Care, and Empowerment

The pathologizing way patients' bodies are described contributes to the apparent normalcy of these surgical transformations, as extreme as they are. In many episodes, we hear of the psychological pain of ugliness or defect, and how cosmetic medicine can contribute to healing and personal wellness. Tess's looks were ruined by pregnancy. Marilynda, a working-class woman from season three who works at Walmart, just wants to fix her broken front teeth and get her smile back. Jeffrey, a formerly obese man, now looks freakish because of the excess skin that hangs from his body. Similarly, the show describes Elisa, Tim, Angela, and Amy as having been tortured by their scarred, ruined, or homely looks:

> If beauty has an alma mater, it's at Beverly Hills high school, the inspiration for the TV show *Beverly Hills 90210*. But the zip code brings back bad memories for Elisa . . . whose appearance caused her to be the brunt of ridicule and alienation.

> After years of torture from classmates, Tim, a thirty year-old assembler for Siemens Energy and father of two from Kenton, Ohio, wanted a new look to match his improved self-esteem.

> Angela has preferred to stay at home rather than socialize because of her looks. All her life she endured constant torment due to her "cartoon character" appearance.

> Amy's deep scars from acne have not only scarred her face, but her life as well. They are a constant reminder of times that she would rather forget. The Extreme Team helps to restore both her beauty and self esteem in this incredible transformation.[9]

Extreme Makeover describes the abject body as a source of deep, life-wrecking, sometimes even disabling distress. For people so cursed, cosmetic surgery is a miraculous resource. When it brings an end to constant torment, allows a person to socialize more freely, or buttresses a person's self-esteem, cosmetic surgery is not a practice of indulgence, misrepresentation, or experimentalism, but rather one of self-care.

When cosmetic surgery patients describe themselves as just wanting to be normal, they affirm socially acceptable reasons for cosmetic surgery, as Kathy Davis found in her study of female cosmetic surgery patients. As I elaborate in the next chapter, Davis argued that women want cosmetic surgery not to be more beautiful, but rather to be more normal. Cosmetic surgery is about identity, argues Davis, not simply vanity. Yet, even though they insist on normalcy, Davis says that sometimes women also "acknowledge that beauty did matter to them."[10] There is a tension between ideas of normalcy—of just wanting to be ordinary—and of beauty, of wanting to fulfill the "dream," as *Extreme Makeover* puts it, of being special and ideal. In my reading of *EM*, the show is selling the dream of beauty, not just normalcy—at one point, for example, Marilynda is described as the "sleeping beauty" as she is anesthetized for surgery, and later the narrator says that the team of doctors has "awakened the sleeping beauty within" her.

A clear distinction between normalcy and beauty is hard to make for *Extreme Makeover* because *EM*'s "ideology posits normalcy as synonymous with beauty," as Brenda Weber puts it in her critical essay on *EM*. And "since it is clearly more normal to be 'plain' than to be beautiful, we have to wonder just how coveted normalcy is."[11] But ultimately, whether they achieve normalcy, beauty, or both, all of the cosmetic surgery makeovers on the show are presented in terms of cosmetic wellness. The participants are presented as enacting agency and self-care in refashioning their bodies. In presenting their version of cosmetic well-ness, these narratives sometimes borrow a self-care dis-course from liberal feminism. The women, in particular, are presented as finally demanding what they are really en-titled to. As Stacey tells the camera during her appoint-ment with the hair stylist, "I've never been pampered and I'm loving it." She jokes, "I don't want to go home now." And Stephanie tells us that this kind of pampering is some-thing she could never allow herself as a mother. In her words: "I would feel guilty taking money from my chil-dren." She expresses excitement at finally "having some-thing for myself," and we hear the excitement in her voice when she says, "I don't look like a mom anymore!" Her story, then, is that of a woman who embraces the chance to overcome the mundane problems of gendered domestic life. Even her pain is presented in terms of self-care. "It was worth it," she and the other participants say over and over again. Just before being wheeled into surgery, Stephanie de-scribes, "This is my change and I'm going for it. There's no stopping me now." The individualist and therapeutic dis-course of embracing opportunity to help oneself is at work here. In other examples from *EM*:

> Lachele is a twenty-four-year-old care worker for mentally disabled people from Cincinnati, OH, who dreams of one day becoming a nurse. . . . But her looks prevent those around her from taking her seriously and seeing past her appearance. Now Lachele will travel to the "Makeover Mansion" and get a chance to take care of herself, after helping so many others.

> Reclusive housewife Valerie, from Bland, MO, has always shunned interacting with the public because of her appearance and insecurities. Since her mar-riage and raising her four kids . . . Valerie has grown

accustomed to her stay-at-home routine, comfortable in her solitary cooking and cleaning. Now that their teenaged kids are growing up, Valerie would like to see what life is like beyond her white picket fence, and so turns to the Extreme Team to give her the chance to transform from homely to hottie.[12]

Thus not only life-wrecking pathology but even ordinary ugliness and domestic tedium can be a situation that calls for cosmetic surgery. Moreover, to undertake cosmetic surgery is a way out of a life of gendered servitude. Cosmetic surgery is paying positive self-attention and recognizing that one is worth the trouble, and even pain, of self-care. This logic, as Louise Woodstock describes, identifies cosmetic surgery as a resource for personal empowerment for any woman, not just the tragically flawed: "Whereas 30 years ago the cosmetic surgery patient required an operation to address a debilitating insecurity resulting from a physical flaw, today that patient starts out as an empowered woman 'doing it for herself' by making herself feel and look even better after surgery than before."[13]

Of course, this kind of empowerment usually takes a great deal of money. Many of the recipients of extreme makeovers—including a Walmart clerk, nurses' aide, factory worker, and homemaker—are working class, and their surgeries would normally be far out of their financial reach. This is one of the underlying logics of dream-fulfillment in *Extreme Makeover*. The show gives people not only bodies they otherwise could never have imagined but also bodies they never could have imagined paying for themselves. For them, being chosen to be on *Extreme Makeover* is presented as something like winning the lottery. This point was underscored for me by one woman I interviewed, named Lucinda, a mother of five who, like Luke, had a good deal of hanging skin after weight loss. For more than a year after her weight loss, Lucinda had been desperate to find a way to pay for a body tuck. (She described her post-weight-loss arms, for example, as "bat wings.") She told me that she thought about applying to be on *Extreme Makeover* to fund the surgery, even though she thought the experience might be humiliating. "I seriously considered applying for *Extreme Makeovers*," Lucinda told me. "I talked about it with my friend and I was thinking about how crappy it would be to go on national TV and show pictures of myself and my icky body. But I'm seriously considering writing *Extreme Makeovers* again. I'm running out of possibilities. You can only be so creative. . . . [But] it seems like the luck of the draw. I don't want to put my future health in a lottery. It would be like winning the lottery." Lucinda was never accepted for the show, but eventually Lucinda's story has what she sees as a happy ending: after months of pursuing surgeons and her insurance company, she managed to get a surgeon to perform the procedure pro bono. But the story Lucinda tells about trying to "win the lottery," to receive the medical resources that the *EM* participants do, complicates the idea of self-empowerment that is being linked to cosmetic surgery. Thus, there is a contradiction in *EM's* logic: On the one hand, cosmetic surgery is presented as a way of taking action and doing something for oneself; on the other hand, such a makeover is out of reach for most people.

Pain and Risk

Here, extreme cosmetic surgery is coded as a practice of self-care that brings wellness. To this end, cosmetic surgery is regularly stripped of any interpersonal, financial, and physical aspects of surgery that might complicate this view. Most notably, the physical pain and trauma of surgery are, to varying degrees, minimized on this show. As Brenda Weber points out, an hours long procedure becomes two minutes, and a weeks-long recovery becomes five minutes, or much less. As she pointedly writes: "time's manipulation is a critical way of managing pain."[14] That's not to say that there aren't dramatic images of the physical aspects of surgery. The audience is made aware that there is pain involved in many of these procedures, particularly in the early episodes of the show. In Luke, Stacey, and Stephanie's episode, we see them pushed in wheelchairs, their bodies and heads wrapped, and we see swelling, bruising, and blood. They are nervous and afraid. Over and over again, the patients are hugged and their hands are held by the surgeons and nurses. Dr. Fisher reminds one patient before her operation, "We're going to take good care of you." The patients are taken after their operations to a "luxurious after-care facility" where they recover—surely not the experience of most cosmetic surgery patients, many of whom get their surgeries as outpatients in ambulatory clinics. Even so, their experiences don't look like much fun. Luke, for example, can't even get out of bed after his abdominoplasty, and the women, wrapped in bandages, look "weird," as Luke put it, with their heads and faces covered in plastic and gauze. The pain and recovery processes are given (limited) airing, yet because cosmetic surgery is presented as a personal accomplishment and a form of self-care, the physical downsides of cosmetic surgery are framed primarily as obstacles to be overcome. As Stephanie says, interviewed in her wheelchair and bandages, "We're all going through a whole lot right now. We don't feel good but it's all going to be worth it in the end." Over and over again, we hear the refrain that the pain is "worth it." In other episodes, especially in the second and third seasons of the show, the pain, trauma, healing, and recovery involved in surgery are barely mentioned. Marilynda's story, for example, was told in season three without any attention at all to her physical pain or recovery. Having undergone multiple surgeries of the face and body, as well as multiple root canals, tooth extractions, and veneers, Marilynda surely would have had a lot of pain and considerable recovery time, but her story moved quickly from procedure to procedure to the "Big Reveal," the moment where she meets her astonished, impressed family and friends looking like a Hollywood star.

This aspect of *Extreme Makeover* was pointed out to me by some of the cosmetic surgery patients I interviewed. They wondered whether *EM* presented realistic images of the actual experience of getting cosmetic surgery. One woman, a grandmother from California named Deborah who had undergone nine hours of surgery for her own makeover, suggested: "Usually it [the television show] switches from the day of the surgery to four weeks later. They skip all that recovery time. If I would have known I would never have had that done. I had no idea being bound [by the bandages] like that would affect me. . . . The down time—I have a family and a home, there's a lot of things I need to do. I wasn't going to go out the way I was. . . . I didn't go to the grocery store or anything. You're so burned, burning the whole layers of skin off. You're just raw, just completely raw." Deborah described her experience with cosmetic surgery as much more physically difficult than *EM* would suggest. She believed that its portrayal of cosmetic surgery played a role in creating unrealistic expectations for surgery—that she would recover quickly, that the healing would be relatively easy, and that the interruption to her familial and social life would not be prolonged.

Similarly, Michelle, a forty-something cosmetic surgery patient whom I interviewed, sees the show's portrayal of the physical experiences of cosmetic surgery as a kind of "deceptive marketing." Having undergone her own surgical makeover just six weeks before our interview, she saw *Extreme Makeover*'s depiction of surgery as disingenuous: "You see someone for ten seconds saying it's painful, but you don't see it for ten days. For me, the pain was numbing. I had intense pain for three days. I was black and blue for four weeks, and [six weeks later] I still have a little bruising. It's not realistic—it doesn't show the pain or the person interviewed six months later, doing their own hair and makeup, eating the same way they did before. Even the liposuction—what are the repercussions of that?" Michelle's own surgeries might have been chronicled on *Extreme Makeover*: in one surgical session, she underwent a forehead lift, an anterior face lift, upper and lower blepharoplasty (eyelids), a chemical peel and hyaluronic acid injections to plump her lips. However, the procedures were much more painful than she expected, and the results did not please her. She still has a visible incision underneath one of her eyes. In her experience, the pain of the cosmetic surgery makeover was "indescribable," and the other costs—the time off of work, the trauma to her skin, the scarring, the risks, and the many thousands of dollars—were great enough to make her regret her decision: "I'm not opposed to cosmetic surgery, but for me, I'm finished."

Michelle also wondered whether or not the results of *Extreme Makeover* are really as impressive as the show suggests. Do the shows realistically display the effects of cosmetic surgery, or do they exaggerate its effectiveness? The "Big Reveal," the moment where the made-over persons reunite with friends and family, presents a fantastic version of cosmetic surgery. Marilynda, the Walmart

worker, stepping out of a stretch limousine for her Big
Reveal, is described as "sparkly as a diamond"—and, in fact,
is wearing a borrowed Harry Winston diamond necklace
worth half a million dollars. The importance with which
her Reveal is touted almost overtakes the rest of the narrative, as if the moment of showing herself transformed becomes the whole point of the makeover. Even the surgeon
says to her, "you're going to have a *great* Big Reveal!" And
she does. At the event, as they always do, her family and
friends stand in awe, clapping and crying at the amazing
transformation they see. What is this Reveal meant to suggest, aside from the success of the physical transformation?
It is a Hollywood ending, and thus we might expect that
Marilynda's future will be, somehow, fit for such a story. If
EM logic is right, her ordinary life will be vastly made
over. It is hard to imagine that she will go back to her job at
Walmart.

For the most part, the stories told on *Extreme Makeover* often mute or silence the negative aspects of cosmetic
surgery. With the notable exception of two episodes featur-
ing a man named Jeffrey Cooper, to which I will return
later, *EM* largely tells an optimistic, and essentialist, narrative about cosmetic surgery in its first three seasons. In
sum, as I read it, the show produces the cosmetic surgery
patient as a true self that is revealed, honored, or expressed
through cosmetic surgery. In addition, she or he is a suffering self, one who passively and gratefully accepts the
help of cosmetic medicine, while paradoxically also pursuing empowerment. She is not only undertaking a transformation of her body, but of her whole life. She aims for
normative goals of heterosexual partnership, of liberal self-
assertion, of personal self-help. Cosmetic surgery here is a
form of identity work that establishes the true self and the
proper body to reflect it.

Television, Advertising, and Medicine

Extreme Makeover was produced with the complicity and participation of one of the most prominent organizations of plastic surgeons, the American Society of Plastic Surgery. The reason is unsurprising: they thought the show would be good for business. In 2003, the society, which represents surgeons certified by the American Board of Plastic Surgery, held an impassioned debate on *Extreme Makeover*. Dr. Garth Fisher, who is one of the society's members, had participated in a pilot for *Extreme Makeover* and later become one of its primary surgeons. Because the ASPS forbids its members to take part in contests, the issue was put before the ethics committee, which was charged to decide whether or not surgeons who were members of the ASPS could participate. The society's ethics code identified a problem posed by *EM*'s contest: somebody who didn't need cosmetic surgery might win and undergo it unnecessarily. After much debate, which included the resignation of a prestigious member of the ASPS (the president of the American Board of Medical Specialities), the society decided to endorse its members' participation, effectively aligning itself with the show.

The endorsement involved some compromises by *Extreme Makeover*: the show would pay only standard fees to participating physicians, to deter surgeons from making bad decisions because of the lure of extraordinary payment. In addition, physicians maintained final say over whom they would operate on. And, as the *Wall Street Journal* reported, "they also asked that the show plug ASPS and a sister organization, the American Society for Aesthetic Plastic Surgery, Inc., prominently."[15] Even so, the decision to condone their members' participation on *Extreme Makeover* was fraught with controversy within the society. One

ASPS member, Dr. James McCullen, a New England plastic surgeon who specializes in body contouring, described to me his view of the debates: "It was a heated debate on both sides. Ultimately the board voted its approval. . . . I think this could be real positive for cosmetic surgery. It shows us in a positive light rather than something that's totally frivolous. The people they pick aren't frivolous. They're very self-conscious about their appearance. . . . I voted for approval of *Extreme Makeover*, understanding that the downside would be local spin-offs that don't even ask for approval from an ethics committee, or that don't even use cosmetic surgeons to do the procedures."

A few months after the airing of the first *Extreme Makeover*, the ASPS held its annual meeting in San Diego. The society convened a panel to discuss ethical issues in plastic surgery related to reality television. An ASPS press release describes how the televisual production of cosmetic surgery's meanings may conflict with those of surgeons themselves, although like Dr. McCullen, it also views the media opportunistically. According to its press release, there are "potential ethical dilemmas that can arise from advising those shows." Further, "while the plastic surgery community should not hide from such opportunities, individual physicians should always refer to the ASPS Code of Ethics to be sure they are making the right decisions."[16]

The financial incentive of doctors to allow their work to be exploited for television ratings appears significant. There were on average over seven million viewers of the show per week in the 2004 season. In that year, according the ASPS, after having seen a slump, cosmetic surgery "rebounded with a 32% increase in the number of cosmetic procedures performed."[17] The American Academy of Facial Plastic and Reconstructive Surgery, another society of plastic surgeons, put out a press release touting a 22 percent increase in the number of procedures they performed.[18] Initially, the ASPS openly attributed at least some of the growth to television exposure. In its annual report on cosmetic surgery statistics for 2003, the ASPS acknowledged that: "The number of surgical procedures grew by five percent, while minimally invasive procedures jumped 41 percent over 2002." Further, the society suggested that "this past year's growth may be attributed to the attention plastic surgery received from the entertainment industry, which spotlighted plastic surgery and perhaps, created a larger interest from the public."[19] Likewise, all of the surgeons I interviewed readily attributed the recent boom in cosmetic surgery to this media exposure. As Dr. Gellar, an ophthalmologist who performs cosmetic surgery in Florida, told me: "It's basically generalized marketing, raising interest in cosmetic surgery. It's good for us."

Yet by 2005, the ASPS distanced itself from reality TV. In only two years, cosmetic surgery television had become hugely popular, while newspapers were warning of a significant rise in the numbers of people getting cosmetic surgery, raising fears of surgical excess. Even though the link between the cosmetic surgery boom and cosmetic surgery television seemed apparent to many, in its 2005 annual report of cosmetic surgery statistics, the ASPS explicitly denied such a link. The society argued that "Reality TV shows are creating a greater public awareness of cosmetic surgery and may attribute to the growth in procedures; however, these shows have not caused a rampant increase . . . there is no evidence in the statistics to support that TV programs have led to a dramatic surge in the amount of cosmetic surgery procedures."[20] In another press release in February 2005, the society challenged the idea that we are experiencing a cosmetic surgery epidemic due to television exposure: "Many parents worry about the potential influence the media may have on their children's self-esteem and body image. Stories about young women having excessive plastic surgery are enough to keep any parent up at night. However, according to a study published in the March issue of *Plastic and Reconstructive Surgery* . . . only 5 percent of college-age women have actually had cosmetic surgery."[21]

That the society made explicit efforts to dampen the perception that *Extreme Makeover* and other shows had been responsible for a major cosmetic surgery boom reflects the rising perception of excessive cosmetic surgery as a social problem. Surgeons I interviewed agree that in some respects television's celebration of cosmetic surgery promotes unrealistic expectations on the part of patients; according to some, it also promotes the kinds of surgeries the ASPS would call "excessive." Dr. Gellar, for instance, describes cosmetic surgery television as creating absurd or highly unrealistic expectations and promoting too many procedures for each patient. As she told me: "We're so barraged. Cosmetic surgery's on *Oprah, Extreme Makeover.* . . . I've seen *Extreme Makeover* maybe three times. . . . I don't think it's doing a huge service. It justifies things that are over the top. It scares me when I see these young people getting so much surgery. . . . That's courtesy of these shows." Similarly, Dr. Bartholomew, an ear, nose, and throat specialist and cosmetic surgeon who practices in the Northeast, described to me how *Extreme Makeover* and other shows foster absurd expectations in his patients: "They are too much pushing for a young look. For slim and beautiful looking. It is many times hurting the patients rather than helping them. It's not realistic or healthy." Dr. Copeland shares this concern, charging that the show fosters desires for extreme cosmetic surgery. As she said in her interview: "People watch *Total Makeover* [sic], and they think you can have a total makeover in one operation. It used to be that people would have one change [and] would be happy. Now, if people don't change everything, they don't think they've done it."

The ASPS agrees. Repeatedly, the ASPS put out press releases to tell the public that television does not present a serious enough picture of cosmetic surgery. The ASPS decided to release a patient "safety kit" which offers information on cosmetic surgery, and has published repeated warnings to potential patients to remember that cosmetic surgery is real surgery: "Plastic surgery is serious and just as with any operation, surgical procedures carry risks. . . . With the increasing popularity of plastic surgery, combined with the reality show *Extreme Makeover*, it could be easy for the general public to overlook the serious nature of elective cosmetic surgical procedures."[22] At its semi-annual meeting in December of 2004, the American Medical Association similarly chastised reality television: "Reality television shows that depict surgery should not minimize the seriousness and risks of surgery and distort patient expectations," the AMA announced in a press release.[23] The AMA called upon reality television shows to operate with the same ethical principles as physicians must follow, clearly acknowledging the risks as well as benefits of surgery.

The ASPS also recognized that, as Dr. McCullen predicted, after *Extreme Makeover*, there would be "local spin-offs that don't even ask for approval from an ethics committee." The ASPS protested the "new wave" of surgery television shows, making specific reference to MTV's *I Want a Famous Face*, where people try to look like their favorite movie stars. The society argued:

"The new wave of plastic surgery reality television is a serious cause for concern," said Rod Rohrich, MD, ASPS president. "Some patients on these shows have unrealistic and, frankly, unhealthy expectations about what plastic surgery can do for them." Plastic surgery should not be viewed as an avenue to transform a person's looks or life, according to Dr. Rohrich. Rather, plastic surgery can help refine and/or improve on someone's natural appearances. Of particular concern to Rohrich is the young impressionable audience watching these shows who are already self-conscious about their body image.[24]

The society also took umbrage at the show *Nip/Tuck*, not a reality show but a drama depicting a Florida plastic surgery center and its surgeons, who are good-looking, arrogant, and melodramatic and often behave badly. (On occasion, for example, they even have sex with their patients.) "[T]he society takes great offense at the spurious depiction of its medical specialty, which is dedicated to restoring and reshaping the human body. While the FX 'drama' of the south Florida plastic surgery center is sensational, bordering on the absurd, it certainly is not realistic."[25] Given the distinctions surgeons themselves are keen to make, it is important to point out that *Nip/Tuck*, *I Want a Famous Face*, and other shows are not homogenous in their depiction of cosmetic surgery. In Brenda Weber's reading, for example, both *Nip/Tuck* and *I Want a Famous Face* are much more critical of cosmetic surgery than *Extreme Makeover*. For example, she argues that *I Want a Famous Face* is so graphic, and so critical of its own participants, each of whom spends his or her own money to try to look like a particular famous person, that it may actually serve as a deterrent to cosmetic surgery. Further research might pursue not only, as Weber does, the different ways television shows portray cosmetic surgery but also the distinct ways cosmetic surgeons have reacted to them. As Dr. McCullen pointed out, *EM* portrays cosmetic surgery in a positive light, and its patients as deserving and not "frivolous." Other shows that do not do this have been the target of particular umbrage from cosmetic surgery societies. Between 2003 and 2006, the society usually refrained from criticizing *Extreme Makeover* directly, but it critiqued *EM*'s competitor shows, drawing distinctions between good and bad surgery practices, qualified and unqualified surgeons, and realistic and unrealistic portrayals of cosmetic surgery.

From the perspective of cosmetic surgeons, TV depictions of cosmetic surgery matter. Despite its claim that cosmetic surgery television should not to be considered the driving engine of the cosmetic surgery boom, the ASPS used its official status on many occasions to try to direct how cosmetic surgery television is being socially received. Having officially approved of the show and having initially been excited by the public response, the society's tone changed. The market value of *EM*'s positive portrayal of cosmetic surgery is apparent. At the same time, cosmetic surgeons have openly worried about the impact of TV on the public's perception of cosmetic surgery, particularly the rise of excessive surgery or surgery addiction. Through its public relations, the society attempted to discursively manage the meanings of cosmetic surgery television toward its preferred interpretation: cosmetic surgery is serious rather than frivolous, surgeons are professionals rather than opportunists, and patients are, or at least should be, healthy and rational people making positive, life-affirming choices.

Conclusion: The Troubling Case of Jeffrey Cooper

The cosmetic surgery that *Extreme Makeover* produces accomplishes a dramatic transformation of the body, but it is normative in its aims. It pathologizes the body in order to claim the psychological wellness of its participants. It produces the true, authentic self of the individual that is affirmed by cosmetic surgery. The sleeping beauty inside of Marilynda, the real woman inside of Stacey, and the indestructible and ethnically authentic spirit of Tess are all affirmed through modifying the body. Through cosmetic surgery, Luke confirms his character, what he stands for; Tim gets a look that matches his improved self-esteem. Cosmetic surgery is a personal accomplishment for each of these people, reflecting their inner will and self-empowerment. And while the makeover may be extreme, the surgeries are not too physically, socially, or interpersonally complicated to interfere with the goal of affirming their identities.

EM discursively produces the cosmetic surgery patient as a sympathetic and ultimately victorious character, and presents positive images of cosmetic surgery and its technologies. This vision of cosmetic surgery is highly profitable for cosmetic surgeons, but according to the ASPS, and to surgeons whom I interviewed, it demands many caveats. In attempting to manage the media message of cosmetic surgery television, surgeons produced their own vision of the cosmetic surgery patient. Good patients have healthy expectations; they must not expect to transform their lives; they must not be overly optimistic about transforming their looks; they should be serious, not frivolous; they should be measured, not extreme. Bad patients want to look like someone else (either metaphorically or literally,

as in *I Want a Famous Face*). They want to drastically
change their looks. They want to transform their lives.
Cosmetic surgeons' own vision of cosmetic surgery, as expressed by societies like the ASPS and the ASAPS, sometimes overlaps with that of *Extreme Makeover*, but also
complicates *EM*'s vision.

But the meanings of *Extreme Makeover* and other TV
shows cannot be contained by the public relations campaigns of cosmetic surgery societies. As Brenda Weber has
pointed out, *extreme makeover* is now a floating signifier—
it is a concept people know, use, appropriate, and apply to
other shows, contexts, and issues. It is also appropriated by
some cosmetic surgeons themselves, who offer their own
versions of the makeover to their patients. Consider the
following advertisement for the services of a cosmetic surgeon, published in *New York* magazine, which unapologet-
ically promotes "extreme makeovers"—not for winners of
a television contest, but for anyone who might be unhappy
with their looks. In the ad, a pretty, smiling woman declares:

> **My Extreme Makeover Changed My Life!**
> If you are at all like me, you are most likely dissatis-
> fied with certain aspects of your face and body. David
> Ostad, M.D., noted Park Avenue surgeon, helped me
> to choose the plastic surgery procedures which best
> suited my needs. I urge you to call and meet Dr.
> Ostad. He'll tell you what surgery is best for you and
> perform it expertly.—Dawn, actual extreme make-
> over patient.[26]

Advertisements like Dr. Ostad's, unthinkable twenty or
even ten years ago, are unremarkable now if we accept the
view of cosmetic surgery presented on the show which inspired it—that an extreme makeover accomplishes a radical

transformation of the body, but it aligns the body with its more real or authentic self. It repairs pathological bodies and promotes cosmetic wellness. And although the makeover may be extreme, the surgeries are not too costly (physically, socially, or otherwise) to interfere with changing one's life for the better.

There are many ways to critique this production of cosmetic surgery's meanings, but here I want to point out that the vision of cosmetic surgery generally promoted by *EM*, and by some cosmetic surgeons, is complicated by one story of cosmetic surgery that appeared on the show itself. The story of Jeffery Cooper suggests that cosmetic surgery can be complex, difficult, and ambiguous in its effects. In conclusion, I briefly explore Jeffrey's story, suggesting that it offers potential fodder for an immanent critique of *EM* and other promotions of cosmetic wellness.

In the first episode where Jeffrey is featured, his physical transformation amazes his friends and family, and his surgical makeover is presented as a success story. However, risks and downsides of his surgery were explored in a special follow-up segment on another episode of *EM*. Like Luke, Jeffery was a formerly obese person who had lost a massive amount of weight through diet and exercise—in this case, an astonishing two hundred pounds. He was left with a great deal of hanging skin—in effect, he was wearing a suit of skin that would fit someone more than twice his size. He described the experience as a "cruel joke" that life played on him. Having worked so hard to lose the weight, he now looked freakish. He was a charity case: the voiceover narrator says that "we decided that he needed our help." In addition to surgeries of the face, nose, teeth, and eyes, he was given an abdominoplasty, a thigh plasty, and a brachioplasty for his upper arms—a triple body tuck—to remove excess skin. The process required three surgeons working at once, who removed over a foot of skin. This was no easy surgery and, in fact, Jeffery endured a "life-threatening loss of blood." His recovery, according to the show, was "long and complicated."

It turns out that there were other problems that are revealed in his post-makeover story. The first was interpersonal. We are shown a photo of Jeffrey and his wife taken before the makeover. They are both obese. After his makeover, they have much less in common physically. Jeffrey's wife admits that she was worried that he would now accept her less, that they would no longer look right together, and that people would stare at them. She wondered: how can she stay a fat person looking the way she does, while her husband looks thin and gorgeous? But Jeffrey rejects these arguments for the camera. He says that he accepts her as she is, and that it is "her decision" to choose to either "do this"—meaning the weight loss and makeover—or not to. In a somber moment of confessional reflexivity, Jeffrey says of his wife, "She is her own soul."

Another problem is a physical one: Jeffrey was left with a great deal of scar tissue from the surgeries. In fact, scars are inevitable in many cosmetic surgeries, especially body lifts and tucks, but this is rarely acknowledged on *EM*. Jeffrey's problem, however, is addressed by a new procedure. Cosmetic laser technology promises to target the red coloring of the scars, thus reducing their prominence. And so this follow-up episode, which chronicles the trials and tribulations of Jeffrey's post-makeover life, becomes a secondary makeover, in which the audience and Jeffrey are presented with the promise of new technology which will help ease the unhappy effects of surgery. In this show, technological advancement is the response to the iatrogenic problems of surgery.

The final problem, however, is much more serious, and

can't be resolved easily. Although Jeffrey lost two hundred pounds through dieting and exercise, he never managed to conquer his problem with compulsive overeating. Before his makeover is even finished, he begins to gain back the weight. *Extreme Makeover* initially describes Jeffrey's problem as medical rather than psychological: "Because of a prescribed high protein diet to fight anemia, he suffers another setback when he gains fifteen pounds."[27] But it turns out that, in fact, he had started secretly overeating while he was getting his makeover. We are told in the follow-up episode that "by the time of his Reveal," unbeknownst to the *Extreme Makeover* team, Jeffrey could "barely fit into his clothes. He had already gained twenty-five pounds." Jeffrey says that while he was getting congratulated by his family and friends, smiling his new Hollywood smile, he had a Hershey bar in his pocket. He was gorging in private, and he says that he felt like a "fraud." "How can I let these people down?" he reports having asked himself. Two months later, he had gained back a total of forty pounds, and within a few months after that, people in his community couldn't believe he was the same person that was made famous by *Extreme Makeover*.

Jeffrey seems to have taken control of his compulsive eating by the time of the follow-up episode. He has gone back to restricting his food intake, he is in group therapy, and has lost most of the regained weight. He is an inspiration to others, we are told. He "represents something to people who know him": that it is possible to overcome serious obstacles. He is asked by a local marathon race to carry the torch for them as a symbol of hard work and meeting difficult challenges. But although he is relieved to have brought his weight and his eating back under control, and has regained the approval and admiration of his friends and neighbors, he makes no promises now about the future.

"The show's not over," he says. "I don't know what will happen next." Jeffrey's refusal to declare himself cured for good is also a refusal to tie up the story in a happy ending. Having already seen failure, Jeffrey acknowledges that maintaining a slim body and managing compulsive behavior can be very difficult.

Jeffrey's story, especially as told in the follow-up episode, is unusual for *Extreme Makeover* in a number of ways. First, the episode addresses something of the familial context of cosmetic surgery. Cosmetic surgery doesn't usually happen in isolation, and it may cause tension and disagreement in families and even communities. In addition, the story of Jeffrey reveals the potential physical risks of cosmetic surgery, including the dangers of the operation, and the adverse effects of cosmetic surgery scars, which are otherwise never mentioned on the show. Finally, by openly acknowledging his eating disorder, the show complicates the idea that the true, authentic self—the right, proper, healthy (and in this case, thin) self—can be revealed through the cosmetic wellness of the outer body. Generally, Jeffrey's story offers a messier tale of surgical transformation usually explored in *EM*, which usually presents tidy, uncomplicated stories with happy endings.

As uneven as *Extreme Makeover* is in favor of positive and normalizing images of cosmetic surgery, the show can be read through the lens of the most complex and discordant aspects of cosmetic surgery it allows us to see. Even though Jeffrey's story is atypical for *EM*, the ups and downs of his makeover suggest that there is be a great deal more to cosmetic surgery than the show often likes to reveal. Cosmetic surgery's straightforward aims, its universal efficacy, and its interpersonal effects are complicated by this narrative. Moreover, as this show can be read to suggest, cosmetic surgery's essential self is now a dilemma instead of fixed truth. Fat or thin? Disciplined or undisciplined? Cured or sick? Finished or unfinished? Better or worse? Deserving or undeserving? Although to my mind, and to the minds of the cosmetic surgeons whom I interviewed, *EM* has largely constituted an unapologetic, aggressive promotion of cosmetic surgery, this story reminds us that cosmetic surgery—and its subjects—are ambiguous, contradictory, and far from fixed in meaning.

3

Miss World, Ms. Ugly

Feminist Debates

While *Extreme Makeover* presents the possibility of whole-body surgical overhauls without a trace of addiction or pathology, many feminists have had difficulty imagining any cosmetic surgery, however major or minor, that is not both pathological and addictive. Most feminist critics of cosmetic surgery have described women's decisions to have cosmetic surgery as instances of patriarchal coercion, and some have argued that all women who get cosmetic surgery are at risk for surgery addiction. Alternative accounts in feminist scholarship, to varying degrees, defend women's choices to get cosmetic surgery as rational expressions of women's agency, and address the narrative work that women do to make their cosmetic surgeries less stigmatized. I want to reconsider the debates in feminism over cosmetic surgery, seeing them as implicated in the construction of the cosmetic surgery subject. I argue that feminist thinking on cosmetic surgery not only needs to move beyond the structure-agency debate but also must be more critical of its own problematizations of cosmetic surgery.

Feminist Fears of "Becoming Surgical"

The "beauty ideals" perspective is the most well-known feminist position on cosmetic surgery. This perspective identifies cosmetic surgery as a particularly heinous outcome of beauty culture. In this view, beauty culture encourages women to compare themselves to impossible standards of attractiveness and disciplines women into spending their time, psychic energy, money, and health trying to achieve them. Oppressive cultural ideals pressure women to think of their bodies as objects, primarily in terms of their sexual appeal to men. Although in many ways similar to other beauty practices, cosmetic surgery, because of its physical risks, permanence, and invasiveness, is seen as one of the ultimate practices of self-harm in beauty culture, used by women who experience self-hatred, insecurity, and an unhealthy desire to please men at their own expense. This perspective indicts cosmetic surgery itself as politically corrupt—as an example of the medicalization of gendered beauty norms—and also perceives women who use the practice as having internalized oppression or false consciousness.

Feminist writing since the 1970s has identified cosmetic surgery with women's deep psychic victimization, and the recent cosmetic surgery boom has drawn renewed concern. One example is Virginia Blum's book *Flesh Wounds: The Culture of Cosmetic Surgery*. Blum begins by describing her own experience of being taken by her mother to a cosmetic surgeon as a teenager. She underwent a rhinoplasty, which gave her a nose that she thought aesthetically terrible, and she describes a years-long ordeal to correct the surgeon's damage. Although Blum's experience seems especially traumatic, she takes the view that hers was not different from other women's experiences. To her mind, any cosmetic surgery is a practice of coercion that preys upon people who are pathologically self-hating. She writes, "Just because culture has normalized our pathology . . . it doesn't mean that cosmetic surgery isn't like any other practice that has us offering up our bodies to the psychical intensities that angrily grip us."[1]

Blum argues that the source of this pathology is celebrity culture, which instills in women a toxic narcissism. She points out that whereas cosmetic surgery once belonged to celebrities, it now belongs to ordinary women as well. Although we once might have left physical perfection for Hollywood stars to pursue, women now see ourselves in hypermediated form. We relate to our bodies as if we, like celebrities, had to constantly worry about forging "particular looks and impressions" for others.[2] "Little by little," she writes, "we are all becoming movies stars—internally framed by a camera eye."[3] In Blum's view, women are not so much driven by the stigma of the ugliness of a particular body part, or even the desire to be ordinary, but rather by the promise of what the body *could* be. "The body is nothing until it's jolted into being by the image of something it could become—a movie star, a supermodel, a beautiful body. It's a body you have only when it's *the* body. Perhaps we want to possess the body we don't have to begin with. Working out, having surgery, just dieting— these are acts that give the body a cultural reality. It's not only the puritanical, subjugated body that submits to the cultural regimes of the beautiful. Rather, we invent regimes as routes toward inventing this body."[4] Thus, theoretically at least, women who feel satisfied with their individual body parts may still desire cosmetic surgery, because it is the very act of transforming the body that gives it social and cultural value.

Although all women are subjected to the toxic effects

of celebrity culture, Blum identifies women who actually undergo cosmetic surgery as particularly sick. In fact, she equates cosmetic surgery patients with people who have delicate self-harm syndrome, a psychiatrically recognized mental illness diagnosed mostly in young women who repeatedly cut themselves. Blum rhetorically asks: "how different is going under the knife in search of youth and beauty from some ritual and hidden adolescent cutting?"[5] That cosmetic surgery is akin to the compulsive behavior of a self-mutilator is not, in her account, hyperbole. Blum sees that surgery addiction "is built into the practice" of getting cosmetic surgery.[6] Once a person becomes surgical, which happens when "surgery enters your world as a remedy for the body's flaws," she will inevitably have more surgery.[7] According to Blum, the media lures women into becoming surgical. Once they do, their unrealistic expectations will ensure they are not satisfied with just one. "Patients cannot and will not accept that cosmetic surgery isn't a miracle. From the wistful expectation that the next surgery will finally correct the disfiguring damage [of a cleft palate] to the wishful thought that it might give you the movie-star level of looks denied you by nature, it's difficult to resign yourself to the mortal limitations the very practice of plastic surgery seems to transcend—at least in our cultural imaginary."[8] Blum insists that cosmetic surgery is not only physically but also psychically dangerous in that it can transform us from ordinary to surgical, from surgical to perversely addicted. She closes her book by warning us that if we have one operation, this will happen to us: "You will look in the mirror, smile back at the image reclaimed, and relish the grace period between this operation and the next one. The beast-flesh will grow back."[9]

This is one of the most powerful charges that feminists now employ against cosmetic surgery: that the practice is addictive, creating surgery addicts or junkies who will inevitably get one surgery after another. In the play *The Good Body*, Eve Ensler presents her version of a cosmetic surgery junkie. Like Ensler's *The Vagina Monologues*, this play is structured as a series of monologues by female characters (all played by Ensler herself, in the production I saw in 2004). Her surgery junkie is based on a thirty-five-year-old model whom she interviewed in Argentina. The model has had many plastic surgeries and has become famous for both the incessant surgeries and for the apparently beautiful results. Ensler presents her character as a spectacular example of a surgery addict. She recites the monologue while lying on the stage floor, covered with a sheet, invoking images of an operating table or a hospital bed. A camera helps us see Ensler's body projected on a screen in front of us, so that our view is as if we are hovering over the hospital bed ourselves. The effect is powerful. When I saw the play in New York, it seemed to me that the whole audience gasped after the model recounts the surgeries she has undergone. The character is shocking because of the sheer scale of her surgical project.

Yet she is also predictable, the epitome of feminist characterizations of cosmetic surgery patients: male-identified, indifferent to her health, and ready to engage in every conceivable kind of surgery to make her man happy. The character tells us that she once liked to have a few glasses of wine, let her hair go unwashed, and sleep until noon. Now, through cosmetic surgery, she has the "confidence to . . . imagine being perfect."[10] This process was initiated by her plastic surgeon. After one operation, he mapped her future operations on a photograph of her body: "There were corrective red marks all over my body like the kind you got on your spelling takes in seventh grade. . . . 'Your body is a map,' he said. 'These red marks are designated beauty capitals that need attention and work.' "[11] Just as Blum foresees, this model could not stop once she started. Six years later, her body has been completely reworked. In fact, she married her plastic surgeon, nicknamed Ham. She is the ultimate sex object, literally created and reshaped by her husband.

> Today I am a Ham creation. I've had lipo on my stomach, butt, and thighs. . . . I have newer Soya implants that do not harden and feel kinder to the touch. That was for Ham. We started dating after he made my tits softer. That really turned him on. He was feeling my breasts all doctorly. Then something changed. It just got different. Before I knew it, Ham had climbed up on top of the operating table and we were doing it. I think how wonderful it must be for him to actually make love to what he's created. . . . Twice he's discovered areas with his fingers and tongue that needed more work. Sometimes I worry what will happen when he runs out of parts of me to change . . . that he'll just get finished and lose interest.[12]

At the moment, however, it seems that there is always the promise of another surgery around the corner.

But what makes this woman such a surgery junkie? Is it a particular kind of patient who is likely to be an addict, or the surgery itself that is an addictive practice? Ensler's characterization of the model was partly an indictment of her character: she spoke like a stereotypical bimbo, in a high voice, giggling and drooling over her husband like a teenager. A number of times the audience laughed during the monologue. This woman was silly. She was shallow, vain, and at least a little bit stupid. She did not just dislike a singular body part but, under the influence of her surgeon, saw her whole body as a zone of improvement and beautification. From this portrayal, we could surmise that the cosmetic surgery junkie is a particularly vulnerable woman, unusually vain, especially male-identified, and self-hating. But Ensler's surgery junkie is situated alongside other narratives in *The Good Body* that describe an array of body practices, from compulsive dieting and exercise to body piercing and Botox, that Ensler sees as harmful to women. Women's bodies are subjected to, as she summarizes it: "sucking, spending, scrubbing, shaving, pumping, pricking, piercing, perming, cutting, covering, lightening, tightening, ironing, lifting, hammering, flattening, waxing, whittling, starving, and ultimately vanishing."[13] For Ensler, cosmetic surgery is only one (albeit one of the worst) of many self-harm practices that women undertake, and addiction to cosmetic surgery represents the extreme end of a condition of self-disgust that most, if not all, women experience. The ultimate message here is, as Ensler pronounces in capital letters in the text version of the play: "LOVE YOUR BODY. STOP FIXING IT."[14]

Blum and Ensler promote radical feminist positions that identify women's bodies and their victimization as primary targets of patriarchy. For them, the body ought to be left alone; women's bodies are only authentic when they are "natural." In these accounts, the body is a passive object. The subject of cosmetic surgery internalizes, and promotes, the objectification of her own body. This view is part of a tradition in feminism that is hostile to beauty practices in general, because they are perceived to be a form of alienated self-objectification. As Liz Frost summarizes: "Women's engagement with their looks is interpreted as imposed by patriarchy for men's gratification, as alienating of the potential alliance of woman with woman, and as a distracting diversion from a woman's real self, located internally. After centuries of looks being seen as reflective of women's personalities, their looks can, within this strand of argument, be interpreted as some kind of external opponent, or even enemy, which may actively hinder women from finding their real selves."[15] A number of feminists, including Kathy Davis, have criticized the dualism of this view. The suggestion that cosmetic surgery modifies the body as a passive object is, for Davis, a false one. For her, practices like cosmetic surgery are expressions of the self's dynamic relation to and with the body. In her account, which I will describe in more detail below, cosmetic surgery is an identity practice that transforms both body and self.

There are other problems with the radical feminist position. As Frost points out, this view employs an essentialist conception of the self. The idea that women's bodies are only authentic when they are left alone, and that body practices deny women's real selves, problematically posits an essential self that precedes lived embodiment. As many critics of radical feminism have argued, essentialist views of the self are homogenizing. They universalize and fix women's subjectivity, and treat cosmetic surgery patients monolithically. In this logic, the surgery that was pressed on Blum as a teenager is no different from the many operations of the Argentinean model, nor different from others' experiences. Cosmetic surgeries are pretty much all the same, and so are the women who get them: to greater or lesser degrees victimized, self-hating, and estranged from their authentic selves.

The Rebellious Feminist Body

There are other critiques of cosmetic surgery within feminism which do not assume a natural body and an authentic self that can be recovered from culture. Following

Michel Foucault, Susan Bordo offers a less essentialist account of how gendered power relations are expressed in women's body practices.[16] Bordo supplements Foucault's description of how power circulates in disciplinary ways, inculcating subjects with norms of self and body, with an account of the gendered relations of such discipline. Women's body practices, Bordo suggests, follow the imperative for self-mastery generally promoted in modern industrialized cultures. The circumstances in which they do this are shaped by a gendered mind-body dualism that locates women closer to corporeality than men, rendering women's fleshliness especially threatening, and by the cultural discourses of femininity, which establish acceptable modes of gendered embodiment and subjectivity. In this context, a practice such as cosmetic surgery can be seen as a disciplinary, gendered expression, but not necessarily one of sick or pathological subjects. Rather than authentic subjects internalizing oppression and becoming inauthentic, women's very subjectivities are shaped, from the start, by these modes of self-relation. Women's bodies are not objects. Instead, they are rather "sites of struggle, where we must work to keep our daily practices in the service of resistance to gender domination, not in the service of docility and gender normalization."[17]

In this view, all of us are now compelled to view the body as malleable material for technologies of the self. There is little or no possibility of living in unmodified bodies, and so the feminist challenge is to use body practices in ways that resist gender normalization. Under these circumstances, Kathryn Pauly Morgan imagines that feminists might resist the political pressures of cosmetic surgery by using it ironically. In her utopian account, Morgan imagines a "Ms. Ugly" pageant, where women compete to create bodies that reject heteronormative standards of beauty. They have wrinkles created instead of erased. They have fat injected instead of suctioned away. In her vision, this is how women might use cosmetic surgery to express agency. They would denaturalize, rather than naturalize, beauty; their parody of beauty pageants would expose the constructedness of body norms. They would see the body as a site of action, rather than of passive inscription and acceptance. And they would highlight the role of technology in shaping women's bodies. Particularly, they would highlight the medicalization of beauty as the "double-pathologizing of women's bodies," since women's bodies have not only been treated as inferior in the histories of medicine but are also being pressured to "achieve [beauty] perfection through technology."[18]

While the prospect of a Ms. Ugly pageant seems unlikely, in one sense its spirit is accomplished in the work of French performance artist Orlan. Orlan uses cosmetic surgery with an overtly intellectual and political interest in provoking us to examine its normative character. Her project, called "The Reincarnation of Saint Orlan" was begun in 1990 and has thus far included twelve cosmetic surgeries. She began by designing her new face digitally, creating a pastiche of iconic images of beauty, combining features of Renaissance paintings, including a brow from Da Vinci's *Mona Lisa* and a chin from Botticelli's *Venus*. After much effort to find surgeons willing to transform her face in an aesthetically anomalous way and in unorthodox conditions, she undertook the surgeries, four in 1990 and the remaining over several years. Each time, she transformed the surgical setting from a sterile, antiseptic operating environment to a performance stage, with props, costumes, and other accoutrements. The surgeries were turned into high-concept performance art, and although she was anesthetized, she spoke during them for as long as possible, sometimes reading aloud while her body was being operated on.

These surgeries have not quite given her the ugliness advocated by Morgan, which would be the mirror opposite of normative beauty ideals, but she has attained a bizarre look that parodies beauty. In fact, at one point Orlan planned a surgery that would create the largest nose that her face can support—a direct reversal of the whole history of rhinoplasty, which in its Anglophilia has created smaller noses. While her performance act has raised charges of self-mutilation and surgery addiction, feminists have largely understood her work as enacting a spectacular, if disturbing, feminist opposition to cosmetic surgery. She is understood as revealing the true, graphic horror of cosmetic surgery that women undertake to achieve beauty ideals. For example, Alyda Faber writes of Orlan that "the artist's use of cosmetic surgery as a medium for artistic expression amplifies the social pressures on women to conform to narrowly defined patriarchal standards of beauty. In fact, her work exposes the violence of these beauty standards insofar as her "reincarnation" project embodies these practices to excess."[19] What Orlan herself has argued, however, is that she wants not to force a rejection of cosmetic surgery but to, in her words, simply "divert plastic surgery from its aim of improvement and rejuvenation."[20] She is not opposed to technological modifications of the body, but only to the norms of beauty that ordinarily inform them: "My work is not against cosmetic surgery, but against the standards of beauty, and the dictates of a dominant ideology, that impress themselves more and more on feminine flesh . . . and masculine flesh."[21] Her work thus endorses the feminist critique of beauty ideals, but it does not assume a radical feminist view of the body as best left "natural," unaltered and unmodified, or a view of body modification as mutilation. Instead, Orlan implies a queer approach to the body and to technology. "I have the skin of an angel but I am a jackal . . . the skin of a crocodile but I am a poodle, the skin of a black person but I am white, the skin of a woman but I am a man; I never have the skin of what I am."[22]

Feminist critics of cosmetic surgery take varying positions on what a feminist response should be. Some, like Virginia Blum and Eve Ensler, imagine cosmetic surgery as always mutilative; the feminist response is to leave the body alone, to "stop fixing it." Morgan, Bordo, and others acknowledge the difficulty of a feminist program to reject technology altogether, and imagine instead ways to turn technology on its head, to use it rebelliously. As I see it, Orlan's version of Ms. Ugly does this, but pushes the critique further to include all bodily norms, including those that impose a straight reading of the body as a natural indicator of the self. In this respect, Orlan's vision is more complex than those offered by Ensler, Blum, and even Morgan. But none of them, Orlan's included, offers an avenue to understand ordinary, beautifying cosmetic surgery as a choice for women, or as an expression of their agency. In contrast, Kathy Davis and others have tried to consider the possibility of women's agency in getting cosmetic surgery. The "agency" feminists, as they have been called, are interested in defending women against charges of being cultural dupes, and in imagining why women might reasonably make the choice to undergo surgery.

Limited Agency, Relative Choice, and Normalcy

Kathy Davis has argued that women who use cosmetic surgery are not simply victims of a male-dominated culture. Uneasy with feminism's monolithic treatment of cosmetic surgery and its patients—its assumption that all cosmetic surgeries and patients are equally oppressive and oppressed—Davis undertook what she describes as a "fem inist balancing act . . . situated on the razor's edge between a feminist critique of the cosmetic surgery craze (along with the ideologies of feminine inferiority which sustain it) and an equally feminist desire to treat women as agents who negotiate their bodies and their lives within the cultural and structural constraints of a gendered social order."[23] This approach was a way for Davis to respond to the "moral dilemma" of "having to take a stand against the practice without blaming the women who take part."[24] To this end, Davis conducted interviews with forty-two female cosmetic surgery patients. She undertook these in the Netherlands, where cosmetic surgery is, under limited circumstances, paid for by the national health insurance. In some cases, she also observed women being interviewed by a health official who would determine whether her problem warranted coverage. Her findings suggest that many women view their own cosmetic surgeries as empowering. Davis finds that, rather than accommodating the desires of the men in their lives, women often make the choice to undergo a rhinoplasty or a face-lift against the wishes of boyfriends or husbands. They see surgery as a positive, self-made choice. Davis herself thinks that cosmetic surgery is a "costly, painful, dangerous, and demeaning practice," but argues that the beauty ideals accounts are "overly deterministic" and treat women like cultural dupes.[25] She finds that women often have what she sees as "credible and justifiable" reasons for cosmetic surgery.[26]

As Davis sees it, one of her most surprising findings is that women who get cosmetic surgery are not especially vain. Davis argues that women who undergo cosmetic surgery are much more interested in feeling normal and in expressing what they see as their real identities than in being gorgeous. In fact, many women she interviewed criticized other women's vanity or concern with beauty. As one of her interviewees put it, "I don't need to be Miss World."[27] Instead, many women identified particular body parts or problems that they found difficult or unbearable, and they saw their own decisions to have cosmetic surgery as a way to correct that problem, rather than to rewrite their appearance altogether. Further, women were often critical of cosmetic surgery in general, and pointed to examples of cosmetic surgery that they thought were pathological, immoral, or unwise.

My own interviews with women cosmetic surgery patients, undertaken at the start of my research for this book, repeated this finding. Lucinda, for example, described which episodes she liked of *Extreme Makeover* by comparing what she thought were the socially acceptable reasons for cosmetic surgery with less acceptable ones: "Lately [on *Extreme Makeover*] they have been getting people whose desires are more legitimate. Some people are getting things that are like, 'Come on! You already look great!' But others, like a cleft chin, it can really make a difference. Anyone who has something that they feel is really terrible about themselves, they should be able to change. That's why there have been advances in medicine." Lucinda, a college-educated mother of five in her thirties, underwent surgeries to firm up the skin after massive weight loss. Like many of the people presented on *Extreme Makeover*, Lucinda sees herself as an ordinary, average-looking middle-class person struggling with her sense of self. Her desire for cosmetic surgery is "legitimate" in her own mind because she does not want a more fabulous, glamorous life than other people, or a body that is exceptional. Rather, she wants to fix an aspect of her body that she feels is both ugly and in contradiction to who she really is. To her mind, there is an ethical hierarchy in cosmetic surgery. Hers is a more ethical aim because it is more closely linked to suffering, to fixing pathology and achieving normalcy.

Another woman I interviewed, Marcia, offered a similarly hierarchical view of the ethics of cosmetic surgery. A middle-aged health-care administrator with grown children, she compares her own reason for getting blepharoplasty to lift her eyelids with the reasons younger women might have: "My surgery has been trying to get back to who I was, not to be something other than myself but to just regain myself. . . . I hate the experience of having in your mind who you are in life, and then not recognizing yourself in the mirror. What I see in the mirror is not who I am in my mind's image. . . . You just want to be back to who you were." But in contrast to middle-aged women who have justifiable reasons for cosmetic surgery, Marcia believes that younger women who get cosmetic surgery may be psychologically unwell: "If you're thirty years old, you have a different agenda. You're trying to be more beautiful. I worry about your sense of self."

For Marcia and Lucinda, good, healthy, and morally acceptable cosmetic surgery is rooted in recovering, reclaiming, or expressing the real self. Bad, unhealthy, or morally suspect cosmetic surgery, on the contrary, would aim to change who one "really" is. For them, as well as for many of Davis's interviewees, cosmetic surgery represents a chance to remove some bodily ugliness or insufficiency which contradicts their senses of self. A too-big nose or too-small breasts or drooping eyelids would be the focus of women's concerns, and correcting the perceived pathology was seen as important for women's sense of self. Cosmetic surgery is not about beauty, then, according to Davis, so much as it is about identity.

Cosmetic surgery is an intervention in identity. It does not definitely resolve the problems of feminine embodiment, enabling a woman to transcend the constraints of her body; nor is it an unproblematic act of liberation. However, by providing a woman with a different starting position, cosmetic surgery can open up the possibility to renegotiate her relationship to her body and sense of self. . . . Cosmetic surgery can provide the impetus for individual women to move from a passive acceptance of herself as nothing but a body to the position of a subject who acts upon the world in and through her body.[28]

As Davis sees it, this directly contradicts the feminist beauty ideals perspective, which argues that women are treating their bodies as objects, rather than themselves as subjects, in getting cosmetic surgery. In these accounts, women are depicted as manipulated, frivolous, and starstruck. In contrast, Davis argues, by treating cosmetic surgery as an intervention in identity, it becomes easier to take women's bodily experiences with gravity, seriousness, and empathy, and to understand how women might see surgery as the best solution under the circumstances. As I see it, there are numerous benefits to this approach, including the fact that it refrains from either essentializing women's bodies and selves or universalizing their experiences. Further, her approach is more likely to create a feminist theory of cosmetic surgery that might actually be recognizable to the women who are her objects of study.

Even for Davis, though, women's cosmetic surgeries take place in the context of enormous suffering. Davis suggests that although women who get cosmetic surgery may not hate their whole bodies or themselves, they are deeply ashamed of specific body parts. In this sense, while

Davis's defense of the rationality of cosmetic surgery patients has irritated some feminists, it is hardly a resounding embrace of the mental health of female cosmetic surgery patients. Women aren't dupes, according to Davis, but this "does not mean that I 'condone' the practice," she writes, "let alone the cultural norms that make women hate their bodies and want to have them altered."[29] As she summarizes, "Cosmetic surgery can enable some women to alleviate unbearable suffering, reappropriate formerly hated bodies, and reenter the mundane world of femininity where beauty problems are routine and—at least to some extent—manageable."[30] The decision to have cosmetic surgery is often part of a "trajectory of suffering," Davis suggests. When a woman becomes concerned with her body, she experiences a downward spiral of "hopelessness, despair, and finally, resignation," and ultimately, her body "becomes a prison from which there is no escape" except through cosmetic surgery.[31] This situation limits women's agency, but it also makes their decisions to get cosmetic surgery more understandable.

In Davis's interviews in *Reshaping the Female Body*, first published in 1995, women were eager to identify their own desires as normal, while readily seeing others' use of cosmetic surgery as potentially pathological. Women also identified cosmetic surgery as a way not only to fix a physical pathology but also promote an authentic, essentialized version of the self. In fact, their accounts often paralleled the logic of cosmetic surgery promoted by *Extreme Makeover*: cosmetic surgeries fixed broken relationships between the body and self, where the "real" self came through by correcting the body. The reparations of cosmetic surgery then amounted to self-care, which in contrast to other people's use of cosmetic surgery, would be a form of empowerment. Debra Gimlin, in her interview account of women who do "body work," from hair styling to cosmetic surgery, found similar logic. She found this politically unsettling. "Far more than the other women I studied," she argued, "the women who undergo plastic surgery help to reproduce the worst aspects of the beauty culture, not so much through the act of surgery itself as through their ideological efforts to restore appearance as an indicator of character."[32]

Why do women describe their own cosmetic surgery in such ways? Davis admits that her interviewees may be strategic in presenting their own cosmetic surgery narratives in order to render them less objectionable to others. (Specifically, because many of her interviewees were attempting to get coverage from national health insurance, they may have felt the need to emphasize their suffering.) Similarly, Gimlin points out that the twenty women she interviewed were "working hard to justify themselves."[33] In particular, women must "deal with the taint of inauthenticity these procedures imply. Although the body appears more normal, the character becomes suspect, with the self, by implication, becoming deviant. The unacceptable act of cosmetic surgery displaces the normative body as an indicator of character."[34] As Liz Frost describes, women feel pressured to normalize their practices in the face of social criticism. In her attempts to conduct group interviews with women about their body practices, she suspected that the taboos against vanity and engagement with appearance played a major role in shaping the narratives women told. "Vanity is unacceptable," she argues, while "self-criticism and discontent" are "the only available position women can take in relation to their own looks."[35] I would argue that this is especially the case with cosmetic surgery, which is often seen as the most extreme body practice women undertake. As Rebecca Wepsic

Ancheta puts it, "Cosmetic surgery, by its very nature, requires some explanation. It is the act of taking a healthy body and causing harm for the sake of surgically altering appearance. The need for explanation increases within a feminist sociopolitical belief system."[36]

To understand this further, Ancheta employed discourse analysis to discover the "rules" that women employ when talking about their cosmetic surgeries. What Ancheta finds in her interviews of twenty-one cosmetic surgery patients is that they employ two rules in their narrations of cosmetic surgery. First, they minimize cosmetic surgery's more difficult aspects, including the pain, physical suffering, and recovery. They refer to "little" cuts, or easy recoveries, or "great" experiences. According to Ancheta, "By minimizing the extent of surgery, research participants avoided discussion of the severity of surgery. . . . Because cosmetic surgery may appear severe to people who are outside the surgery arena, telling minimizing stories is an important way to negotiate the deviance and horror associated with surgery. Communicating their surgery stories as 'normal' takes the edge off the deviance and horror of cosmetic surgery, thereby socially placing cosmetic surgery—and the research participants' socially communicated selves—in an acceptable light."[37] The second rule that they employ is that of self-authorization, represented by the phrase "I did it for myself." The women insisted that no one encouraged them to get cosmetic surgery, nor were they were pressured by the desire to please others. For example, Emily, a thirty-four-year-old woman, said that: "I'm doing it for myself, you know. I feel better about myself. This is who I want to be. This is the way I want other people to see me."[38] Ancheta points out that such an insistence on one's personal agency is important not only to defend oneself against critics but also to prove to her surgeon that she is a good candidate for cosmetic surgery: "From the patients' perspectives, women are trying to be 'good patients' by upholding and subscribing to the 'doing it for myself' rule."[39]

This creates another dilemma of research on cosmetic surgery, one which perplexed me from the beginning of my research for this book. This is not the moral dilemma that Davis describes, of how to be critical of cosmetic surgery without being critical of women. Rather, it is an epistemological dilemma. When interrogated, women who get cosmetic surgery may say that they hate their bodies, that they suffer, or they might say that they are empowering themselves, that they think their own choices are positive and self-caring. In whichever case, what do women's narratives tell us about cosmetic surgery? How should women's narratives about their own body practices be taken? Davis takes them "at their word," as evidence of their agency— their rational, strategic negotiations—in the context of their suffering. While she rejects the idea that cosmetic surgery patients are dupes, Gimlin takes women's narratives as evidence of their need to justify themselves, even at the cost of being politically conservative. Ancheta sees in women's narratives a complex grappling with the stigma, pathologization, and social judgment of others. Radical feminists, of course, would take any of their responses as evidence of women's internalized oppression and false consciousness.

As much as it is problematic to treat women as cultural dupes, to paint a monolithic picture of victimization, and to imply a proper feminist consciousness as the antidote to a false one, it is also difficult to take women at their word. Even though I see Davis's work as overcoming the problems of radical feminist accounts, I also worry that the agency side of the structure-versus-agency debate is just as limited. As Judith Butler warned in *Bodies that Matter*, an intentionist view of the subject as one who wholly determines the meaning of her body practices is problematic.[40] In Butler's view, although gender is not fixed, but instead performative and malleable, we do not individually author the entire meanings of our practices through our intentionality. Applied to cosmetic surgery, we might say that a woman may intend for her cosmetic surgery to express self-care, or, alternatively, to express rebellion, but how she comes to that narrative involves much more than her own consciousness. Instead, the narrative develops as part of and in response to the social and interactive meanings created in the social context for cosmetic surgery. Thus, this dilemma is not easily resolved within the debate over women as dupes or agents, which in Ancheta's terms "oversimplify and polarize" the matter.[41] Feminist thinking needs to move beyond debating the agency of the individual subject, beyond interrogating what she means, whether she intends to be Miss World or even Ms. Ugly.

As I read them, one of the most illuminating directions that the interview accounts of Davis, Gimlin, Ancheta, and Frost point to, but elaborate to varying degrees, is the intersubjective meanings of body practices. I read their accounts as suggesting in various ways that the meanings are produced within the very acts of doing them, making sense of them, accounting for them, and narrating their meanings, all of which happen in a social and interactive context. As Acheta puts it, the meanings of cosmetic surgery "are constructed through the practices of cosmetic surgery and the meanings and interpretations attached to those practices by the women."[42] I would add that the meanings and experiences of cosmetic surgery are also constructed through the interpretations attached to those practices by *others*—by doctors, feminists, the media, and so on—and the interrelations of these. Women's narratives of their own cosmetic surgeries—specifically, the ways they rationalize, justify, or defend cosmetic surgery, or try to be good patients—do not point just to themselves but also to the social pressures women feel to make sense of their practices. They suggest ways in which women struggle with, navigate, and negotiate the meanings—not all on their own, not simply struggling with "moral contradictions," as Davis puts it—but with and against other discourses that have been interested in defining the cosmetic surgery patient.[43] As I see it, these pressures play a significant role in the symbolic interactions that construct cosmetic surgery's meanings.

Emerging work in feminist scholarship on cosmetic surgery is creating an increasingly nuanced picture of this aspect of cosmetic surgery. Debra Gimlin's most recent work, for example, foregrounds the problem of narration and intersubjectivity by exploring cosmetic surgery cross-culturally.[44] If the meanings of cosmetic surgery are intersubjective, and if narrative strategies are created in part by the pressures surrounding women to justify their cosmetic surgeries, then how do women in different cultural and medical contexts differently speak about them? Interviewing forty women in the U.K. who have undergone cosmetic surgery, Gimlin sees much overlap with U.S. interview accounts, but also many differences. For example, she argues that U.S. women are more likely to use language that emphasizes autonomy, individualism, investment, and opportunity. They repeat that they have made this choice for themselves; that they have earned their right to cosmetic surgery by trying other options first, losing weight on their own, and so on. They frankly describe the economy of appearance—how much looking old costs—as well as the costs and financial difficulties of undergoing surgery. And they speak in terms of leveling the competitive playing field, both in the workplace and in the mating markets. In contrast, according to Gimlin, women in the U.K. are more likely to emphasize the trauma of living in a non-normal body. They present medicalized accounts of appearance more readily, embracing the pathologization of particular body parts as a way of explaining how cosmetic surgery became a reasonable choice for them. They emphasize suffering more than opportunity, psychological pain more than empowerment. And in stark contrast to U.S. accounts, women in the U.K are more likely to describe the influence of others—husbands, boyfriends—in their decision making.

Gimlin's interpretation of these differences is that the medical institutional context of each place—a nationalized health care system in one and a free or mixed market one in the other—situates the women very differently in terms of how their decisions for cosmetic surgery are both produced and received. The context of a nationalized health service that in many ways places the patient as a "recipient" necessitates a different kind of rationale for access to medical resources than does a context of private market medicine that places her as a consumer. Even though the national health service in the U.K. may not literally pay for the procedures, for Gimlin the point is that the cultural effects of such a health system in the U.K. creates a different health culture, one of recipients rather than consumers. The extent to which the institutional culture of medicine shapes women's lived experiences and narrations of cosmetic surgery, and the extent to which broader cultural issues are at work, such as ideas of gender, citizenship, victimization, therapy culture, individualism, and so on, are hard to sort out. But in any event, the approach Gimlin takes here, I think, speaks strongly of the intersubjective character of the meanings of body projects, and offers one example of how to try to grasp its complexities.

Other writers are pursuing intersubjectivity through displacing the subject of cosmetic surgery altogether. Nikki Sullivan's work on Michael Jackson, addressed in chapter 1, asks us to look at the multiple ways in which the meanings of his surgeries are produced by discourses outside of his own subjectivity, as well as the relation between those and himself.[45] Meredith Jones is looking at cosmetic surgery through the lens of actor-network theory, which displaces the patient as the center of inquiry, and positions her as only one of multiple "actors," including the surgeon, the technologies, the media, and other aspects of cosmetic culture. For her, the world of cosmetic surgery is one "where agency is negotiated and movable through doctor-patient relationships and interactions, where human and non-human players such as Botox® have roles of high importance."[46] This approach recognizes how complex cosmetic surgery culture is, and how human subjects are situated as part of a whole network of forces with which they interact, but which they do not necessarily control. In addition, Suzanne Fraser has examined cosmetic surgery through medical writings, women's magazines, regulatory materials, and also feminist texts. She has argued that all of these share, in one way or another, essentialist references to "nature," as well as an individualist focus on agency.[47] She is aiming to shift "the object of analysis from the 'true' interior of the subject to the ideological and political implications of the subject's use of language."[48] This approach has ideological and epistemological advantages.

> The recognition that the subject is not only culturally produced in very complex ways but is fleeting and fragmentary, is crucial for a politics that seeks to

avoid a reification of the subject that can occur even where "cultural construction" is assumed. The cultural subject, reconsidered, does not exercise an internalised or possessed agency; rather, he or she is produced through those forms of agency available in culture at any given moment. This is particularly apparent in the case of cosmetic surgery, where forms of agency vary significantly in terms of availability and efficacy across different contexts.[49]

This analysis, along with those of Gimlin, Jones, and Sullivan, are examples of approaches to cosmetic surgery that orient us differently, away from the structure-agency debate, and away from a fixed human subject—usually the female cosmetic surgery patient—as the center of analysis.

Beyond a Moral Dilemma

The subjectivity of women cosmetic surgery patients has not only been interrogated but also produced by feminist modes of inquiry. Take, for example, the spectacle of the surgery junkie created in *The Good Body*. The audience members of Ensler's play openly laughed at the Argentinian model who married her cosmetic surgeon, probably because they agreed with Ensler's ideological message. Not only is the practice of cosmetic surgery objectionable, but so are the women themselves. Apparently, for most of the audience, Ensler's political critique made sense. But I was offended by Ensler's portrayal of the model as a self-hating bimbo. I could not understand why cosmetic surgery patients could be so easily the objects of public ridicule, and why Ensler and other feminists were moved to represent the cosmetic surgery patient in such ways. Kathy Davis describes a similar experience at a feminist conference ten years earlier. According to her account, Kathryn Pauly Morgan gave a lecture that described women who get cosmetic surgery as "Stepford Wives." The audience laughed at the comparison to the 1970s characters—mindless, self-sacrificing women who literally turn out to be male-created robots. Davis felt that the whole audience was with Morgan; they seemed to collectively condemn women who get cosmetic surgery. Davis left the conference wondering about the "gap between us and them, between feminists who openly disapprove of cosmetic surgery and those who either desire it or are willing to support women who do so."[50]

To my mind, these stories do not simply illuminate the gap within feminism. They also implicate feminism itself. Feminist modes of inquiry do not just reveal the cosmetic surgery patient's subjectivity but also produce it in epistemologically specific and morally positioned ways. This begins with what Suzanne Fraser calls feminism's "common reflex" with psychology, psychiatry, and medicine in focusing on the meaning of cosmetic surgery as "inhering in the individual."[51] Radical feminist treatments of cosmetic surgery such as Ensler's echo those of psychiatry and psychoanalysis, which historically have linked vanity and narcissism to women's psychological weaknesses.[52] The ensuing debates over women's agency are also problematic, even when they defend women against charges of mental weakness, because they still turn on questions of the subject: Is she sick, or healthy? Is she victimized, or empowered? Who is the cosmetic surgery patient, and how might her identity account for cosmetic surgery? In pursuing this line of inquiry, feminist debates operate as processes of subjectivation, taking as a freestanding reality the subject which is in the process of being produced. I believe that the moral dilemma set up in feminism, which for years has revolved around the structure-agency debate, is an

unacceptable response to cosmetic surgery, both epistemologically and politically. The pursuit of the subject of
cosmetic surgery fixes her interiority, thus denying the
ways in which becoming, and being, a cosmetic surgery
patient is an intersubjective process influenced by power
relations. Moreover, the interrogation of the character—the
political and mental health—of individual selves does not
challenge, but rather affirms, the processes of subjectivation upon which cosmetic surgery culture depends. On all
sides, the psychic significance of cosmetic surgery is being
scripted. Women are being sold cosmetic surgery on the
basis of its deep psychic meaning and its role in shaping
identity and self-esteem. At the same time, as I describe in
the next chapter, women who undergo cosmetic surgery
are being subjected to new forms of pathologization that interrogate their mental health and contribute to the medicalization of women's concerns with their appearance.
Feminist thinking on cosmetic surgery must consider these
processes of subjectivation more critically. We must refuse
a moral dilemma whose solution depends upon playing
what Foucault called "truth games" over women's subjectivity. We must, as a new wave of feminist scholars are now
doing, acknowledge the complex, intersubjective processes
that create the meanings of cosmetic surgery, while being
self-reflexive about our own role in its power relations.

4

The Medicalization of Surgery Addiction

Many critics of cosmetic surgery have expressed worries that people who undergo it will become hooked, wanting more and more procedures and aiming to look ever more beautiful and young. But what it means to be hooked, and how people get that way, is becoming a matter of public debate. While feminism has identified all cosmetic surgery as problematic and potentially addictive, medical experts—both psychiatrists and cosmetic surgeons—have focused on sorting normal from pathological cosmetic surgery patients. For psychiatrists, the boom in cosmetic surgery represents a new population at risk for Body Dysmorphic Disorder. For cosmetic surgeons, the public awareness about surgery addiction presents significant professional challenges as well as opportunities. In this chapter, I examine the ways these perspectives frame cosmetic surgery addiction, and I address the social and political implications of the emergence of Body Dysmorphic Disorder as the official psychiatric diagnosis for those perceived as surgery addicts.

The Psyche and Cosmetic Surgery

Although surgeons, psychiatrists, and feminist critics see cosmetic surgery very differently, all of their perspectives establish a strong link between the psyche and surgical body modification. They share the idea common to contemporary Western thought that the psyche is revealed on the body's surface. Most of us make similar assumptions. When we see a body undergoing cosmetic surgery, we want to know *why* the person wants cosmetic surgery, and we look deep within the psyche to answer. Many of us believe that there must be reasons for undergoing cosmetic surgery that go deeper than mere aesthetics. To simply be more beautiful we might change our hair color, but we wouldn't actually undergo surgery unless other reasons compelled us. The popular literature on cosmetic surgery urges us to examine these reasons. In her book called *What Your Doctor Can't Tell You about Cosmetic Surgery*, intended as a guide for prospective patients, psychologist Joyce Nash writes, "[S]everal questions should be answered about those bodily features regarded as deficits: How long has this feature been regarded as a deficit? What were the circumstances that caused this feature to be perceived negatively? Was this feature the source of criticism [or] of teasing? Who made this feature the focus of criticism or teasing? What attempts are made to cover up, camouflage, or make up for this perceived deficit?"[1] Nash, like very many observers of cosmetic surgery, is interested in the "amount of psychological pain" that drives people to undergo it.[2]

For some, cosmetic surgery is always a bad choice while for others it is positive, but feminists, psychiatrists, and surgeons all agree that the decision to surgically alter the body is often the result of deep psychological issues. Within much of feminist writing on the subject, the cosmetically surgical body confesses pain of a particularly gendered kind: it suggests an oppressed consciousness in the form of a negative body image. For psychiatrists and psychotherapists, one's body practices are suggestive of one's general psychic wellness, and the decision to have cosmetic surgery is sometimes seen as an indicator of poor self-esteem or other problem. For much of cosmetic surgery's history, surgeons also argued that a patient's desire to have cosmetic surgery is related to psychic pain. This pain is rooted in perceived or real flaws in appearance and in the social pressures people feel to be beautiful or even normal. But surgeons argued that surgery can actually ameliorate individuals' suffering, their poor body image, or inferiority complex. Thus, surgeons were performing a genuine service to their patients.

In the midst of the recent cosmetic surgery explosion, surgeons are less defensive about their field than they once were. There is more public enthusiasm for surgery and a much bigger market for their practices. Surgeons still argue that surgery can help people who suffer because of their appearance—for instance, they might argue that it can help them do better in a competitive work environment, have more self-confidence, and generally enjoy life more—but they don't feel pressure to defend every single rhinoplasty or face lift. As my own surgeon put it to me: "people don't think it's such a big deal anymore." However, cosmetic surgery has newly defined problems brought about by its own popularity. When so many are undergoing cosmetic surgery, and when some are using much more cosmetic surgery than we once imagined possible, we are challenged to develop new medical, social, political, and personal responses. The suffering psyche is still regularly invoked in public debate about these questions. But if not *all* of the new cosmetic surgery patients can be seen as abnormal or dysfunctional, then which ones are? Where do we decide to draw the lines of acceptability? While feminists worry about the beauty culture and the addictive lures of surgical technology, medical professionals are wrestling with new diagnostic criteria designed to help them identify the surgically obsessed.

The Psychiatric Diagnosis for Cosmetic Surgery Addiction

In the mid-twentieth century, Freudian psychoanalysis was highly influential in psychotherapeutic views of cosmetic surgery patients. Psychoanalysis assumed that a patient's desire for cosmetic surgery was a symptom of underlying neurosis. As Nash puts it, "from a psychoanalytic perspective, the desire for cosmetic surgery was believed to involve the unconscious displacement of sexual or emotional conflict, or feelings of inferiority, guilt, or poor self-image, onto a body part."[3] Thus cosmetic surgery was often seen as a misguided and fruitless attempt to address troubles of the unconscious mind, which usually were related to one's early relationships with parents. In the 1950s, as Nash describes, psychoanalysis made an automatic link between sexual neurosis, body image, and a desire for surgery. For example, "A 1950 study of 48 patients seeking cosmetic surgery of the nose claimed to find evidence of the sexual significance of the nose. Their results were interpreted to mean that women were seeking 'to gain or obliterate masculine attributes, while for men with homosexual conflicts, rhinoplasty accomplished symbolically a wish for castration.' "[4] Since the surgery clearly could not address the underlying problem, cosmetic surgery was seen as worthless at best (and harmful at worst).

In recent years, however, psychoanalysis has declined in influence. It has been supplanted by the mental disorder model, which "assumes that mental illness or psychopathology underlies the motivation for cosmetic surgery."[5] This perspective does not seek to identify unique case histories of neuroses, but instead to fit symptoms into more uniform, diagnosable mental disorders that can be treated. The early history of the mental disorder model was highly biased against cosmetic surgery. Nash has traced how in the 1960s, psychiatric studies linked the majority (between 50 and 80 percent) of cosmetic surgery patients to unhealthy psychiatric diagnoses like personality disorders. However, recent studies find a much lower rate of psychopathology among cosmetic surgery patients. Nash suggests that as the influence of psychoanalysis waned, "improved research methodology characterized by greater scientific rigor has eliminated sources of bias and error" in research on cosmetic surgery patients.[6] (She also suggests that "it is conceivable that more psychologically healthy people are seeking cosmetic surgery.")[7]

Although the mental disorder model would disavow any automatic equation of cosmetic surgery with mental pathology, it still pathologizes cosmetic surgery patients. The evolution of psychiatry as a scientific discipline with standardized diagnostic criteria has expanded its influence in contemporary culture and made it useful for screening cosmetic surgery patients. Cosmetic surgery patients are no longer seen as driven by unconscious Freudian motives, and they aren't prescribed years of analysis on the couch. Instead, they are targeted for screening for mental disorders, which are assumed to be at least partially biological in origin and amenable to pharmacological treatment. The most recent of these is Body Dysmorphic Disorder, which is being popularized as a diagnosis for surgery junkies.

According to Katharine Phillips, one of a handful of psychiatrists most responsible for publicizing Body Dysmorphic Disorder, surgery itself is not addictive, nor is culture primarily to blame for creating surgery addicts. Instead, the problem is that there is an under-recognized mental illness, Body Dysmorphic Disorder, which renders its victims vulnerable to obsession with and addiction to cosmetic surgery. According to Phillips, BDD is a biologically rooted condition, possibly exacerbated by culture and psychological makeup, in which individuals are deeply, pathologically concerned with a perceived bodily flaw. BDD sufferers have a severely distorted body image, and the theory of BDD is sometimes referred to as "body image theory." In the British press, BDD is sometimes called "ugly syndrome," but people diagnosed with BDD, according to its official description, are not concerned about general appearance but rather a very specific body part or parts. The biological origin of BDD, argues Phillips, is suggested by the fact that BDD sufferers primarily find relief with antidepressant medications (specifically SRIs, Seratonin Reuptake Inhibitors). Men and women are equally likely to be diagnosed with BDD, a point that Phillips takes as further evidence that cultural pressures of beauty are not wholly, or even primarily, responsible.

Since 1987, the American Psychiatric Association's diagnostic bible, the Diagnostic and Statistical Manual of Mental Disorders (DSM), has listed Body Dysmorphic Disorder, although many mental health professionals had never heard of it until recently.[8] Three criteria must be met to meet the DSM definition. The first criterion is that the person with BDD is preoccupied by an imagined defect in appearance. If the defect is actually perceivable, it must be slight, and the person's worry about it must be "markedly excessive."[9] For example, one must spend a minimum of one hour per day engaged in BDD rituals, such as examining or camouflaging the perceived flaw. Over one-third of people with BDD, suggests Phillips, actually spend more than three hours in BDD rituals. According to Phillips, approximately one-third of people with BDD will seek surgical assistance. Of those who do seek surgery, over 70 percent will specifically seek rhinoplasty, as concern with the appearance of the nose is one of the most common preoccupations of BDD sufferers. The second criterion is that this preoccupation must cause "clinically significant distress or impairment" in functioning.[10] This means, for example, that it disrupts a person's personal relationships, social life, or employment—that is, it renders at least one important area of one's life less than functional. Phillips gives the examples (among other, less extreme cases) of a woman who quit her job because she couldn't bear to be seen in public, and of a man who became suicidal after six operations on his nose. The third criterion of BDD is that the person's obsession cannot be accounted for by any other diagnosis, such as anorexia.

Diagnostic categories developed within psychiatry often suggest that they might be both "common and abnormal, thus needing medical treatment," as medical sociologist Peter Conrad puts it.[11] The DSM-IV-TR, the 2000 edition of the DSM, states that the prevalence of BDD is unknown.[12] It was nearly unheard of ten years ago, but Phillips and other body image theorists argue that BDD is hard to diagnose and is indeed under-diagnosed, actually affecting 1 to 2 percent of the U.S. population. (This translates into millions of men and women.) Phillips argues in her book *The Broken Mirror* that BDD is not rare.[13] The *Psychiatric Times* argues in an article dedicated to educating psychiatrists about BDD that "due to the secretive nature of BDD patients, it is possible that the prevalence rates are much higher [than the DSM suggests]."[14] Both the DSM and body image theorists suggest that the prevalence of BDD among cosmetic surgery patients is higher than the general population: the DSM-IV-TR estimates that among dermatologic and surgical patients, 6 to 15 percent could have BDD.[15] What accounts for the underreporting of BDD, argues Phillips, is that many surgeons and dermatologists had never heard of it until recently, and BDD sufferers tend to see them rather than psychotherapists for solutions. At the same time, others suggest that BDD is "relatively common" in patients seeking elective surgery, and "one of the most commonly recognized psychiatric illnesses presenting to the dermatologic surgeon."[16] Thus, as psychiatric researchers put it in *European Psychiatry*, "The current challenge is to clearly identify B.D.D. in non-psychiatric settings where patients seek inappropriate care, in order for them to get proper and efficient psychiatric treatment."[17]

Medicalization, or "a way of understanding a broad array of human behaviors and problems" as biological or physiological pathologies, is a powerful conceptual tool for linking psychic pain, body image, and cosmetic surgery.[18] Body Dysmorphic Disorder is now being used to medicalize extreme cases of cosmetic surgery and to establish medical standards for patients' psychological attitudes toward cosmetic surgery. Despite its fairly short history as an official psychiatric disorder, BDD is being called a "clinical buzzword" in the current cosmetic surgery climate. As Phillips and her co-author Raymond Dufresne put it, "In recent years, BDD has gone from being a neglected psychiatric disorder to one that is coming better recognized and understood."[19] This is partly due to the framing of BDD as a social problem in the media, which I describe below, and partly due to the direct appeals psychiatrists have made to dermatologists and cosmetic surgeons to look for signs of

BDD in their patients. Although at this point it is not widely recognized and used, four psychiatrists at the Brown University School of Medicine, including Phillips and Dufresne, have developed a formal screening for BDD and have urged cosmetic surgeons and dermatologists to use it to find patients who may have BDD.[20] They argue that surgeons and dermatologists must try to detect BDD, not least because "patients with body dysmorphic disorder are also often dissatisfied with surgical treatment and may sue, threaten or even become violent toward the treating physician."[21] They argue that "it is better to overdiagnose than to underdiagnose" BDD.[22]

Body Dysmorphic Disorder is not the only diagnosis used to address surgery obsession and addiction, but it is surpassing other ways of describing links between mental illness and cosmetic surgery. In the past fifty years there have been numerous types of problem patients described in the cosmetic surgery, dermatology, and psychiatric and psychotherapy literature. Nash includes those who display Body Dysmorphic Disorder alongside other types of mentally ill patients who seek cosmetic surgery, such as "the surgery addict" and "the insatiable patient." The latter is an old category: a 1967 study in *Plastic and Reconstructive Surgery* on the "Insatiable Cosmetic Surgery Patient," for example, describes the typical "insatiable" patient as male, having low self-esteem, hyposexual, with grandiose ambitions, without meaningful long-term personal relationships, extremely obsessional, and aggressive and litigious.[23] The surgery addict, as Nash sees it, "seeks repeated but different surgeries in an unending quest for physical self-improvement by surgical means."[24] Phillips and Dufresne list many other categories of problem patients and argue that these categories ought to be supplanted by BDD as the proper diagnosis: "The dermatology literature contains many descriptions of patients with BDD, often under such rubrics as dysmorphophobia, dysmorphic syndrome, dermatologic hyopochondriasis, and monosymptomatic hypochondriasis. . . . The surgery literature, too, contains many descriptions of BDD, referring to these patients as having 'minimal deformity,' as 'insatiable' surgery patients, as 'psychologically disturbed' patients, and as 'polysurgery addicts.' "[25] Thus the proponents of BDD use the diagnosis retrospectively, arguing that "it has been described [under other rubrics] for more than a century."[26]

These efforts to establish Body Dysmorphic Disorder as a recognized, legitimate diagnosis for problem cosmetic patients are consistent with Peter Conrad and Joseph Schneider's description of the process of medicalization. Their book *Deviance and Medicalization* describes a five-stage process by which behaviors are medicalized.[27] First, the behaviors are already defined as deviant in the public mind. In the case of BDD, it is not that psychiatrists are attempting to convince people that undergoing cosmetic surgery, or particularly multiple cosmetic surgeries, should be considered abnormal behavior, but rather that the behavior which is already generally seen as suspect can be defined medically. Second, in medical prospecting, the behavior is "discovered" to be linked to some scope of medicine by "describing research that creates such a link."[28] This process is being accomplished with BDD in part through: the collection of case histories of possible BDD patients; the retrospective application of the diagnosis to studies of cosmetic surgery and dermatology patients; current psychiatric research of BDD patients; and efforts to get cosmetic surgeons and dermatologists to identify BDD among patients using new screening techniques developed by psychiatrists. In the third step of medicalization, psychiatrists actively promote "the recognition of the problem in medical terms so that its discovery can be legitimated in the public arena . . . the claim must emerge from the professional literature into a wider public arena."[29] Beyond educating cosmetic surgeons and dermatologists, the general public is a target for the new psychiatric message about BDD. In the fourth and fifth stages, the legitimacy of the claims is secured through medical institutions, courts, and legislation. Ultimately, "once awareness spreads to the general range of medical and mental health practitioners more and more new cases will be identified, increasing the stake that the entire profession has in the designation of the disorders."[30]

Body Dysmorphic Disorder is still in the midst of the medicalizing process. It is already being widely publicized to the general public and is becoming socially problematized through the media's description of BDD as a new crisis in surgery culture. I studied media coverage of cosmetic surgery in the United States and Britain in the past ten years and found that BDD is increasingly linked to the escalation of cosmetic surgery, especially in the past five years. Although relatively few people have actually been diagnosed with BDD, in many media accounts, psychotherapists are asked to speculate on which kinds of cosmetic surgery patients might have BDD. In other articles, surgeons are asked to describe patients whom they suspect have BDD, or journalists themselves pose questions about certain kinds of patients whom they think might have the disorder.

The DSM definition of BDD is often recited in media accounts. Journalists often describe people with BDD as those who suffer from distorted perceptions about their appearance and whose lives are significantly disrupted by their preoccupation with the perceived flaws. However, the disorder is also invoked even when symptoms that meet the diagnostic criteria for the disorder are not apparent. For example, people who simply have had surgeries on multiple body parts are regularly suspected of having BDD in media accounts, whether or not they meet the criteria for BDD. In addition, people for whom appearance is a "minor distraction" are sometimes described as having "mild" BDD, even though the DSM definition demands that a person experience significant distress or impairment in an important area of life functioning due to their appearance concerns. These people are thought to be, like the rest of us, suffering from the effects of beauty culture. In these narratives, the medicalized description of BDD is set alongside the feminist beauty ideals theory of cosmetic surgery. A slippery slope is constructed between vanity—particularly female vanity—and mental illness. Even though according to the psychiatric literature BDD afflicts men and women equally, media accounts regularly link BDD to female vanity and concern with appearance. One gets the impression from reading some of the media accounts that ordinary vain people could find themselves having Body Dysmorphic Disorder if they're not careful. Journalists describe a process whereby individuals, especially women, exposed to the media measure themselves against increasingly impossible standards of beauty and then become addicted to cosmetic surgery. The logic includes arguments such as: "Both temperament and culture contribute to the risk of BDD. . . . The culture reflected in our mass media and advertising emphasizes physical perfection and promotes a favorable view of cosmetic surgery."[31]

In other media descriptions of BDD, people who have spectacularly weird or abnormal tastes, like Jocelyn Wildenstein (the so-called Cat Lady) and Michael Jackson are invoked by journalists and the surgeons they interview as potential BDD sufferers. Unusual aesthetic tastes are problematized, as are unusual surgeries. Seemingly ordinary women who undergo unusual surgeries, like female genital cosmetic surgery, have been described as especially likely candidates for BDD diagnosis. A 2004 newspaper article on genital cosmetic surgery, somewhat humorously titled "Down There, Out There: Women's Procedures Test Limits," describes the procedure as one that appeals to vulnerable, mentally ill women:

> Women who once thought it was enough to have cosmetic surgery to enhance the face, feet and torso now have a new body part to fret about. In surgical suites from the Upper East Side to Queens and the nearby suburbs, women are paying from $3800 to $8000 per procedure to have their genitalia altered. . . . The growing popularity of these cosmetic surgeries has troubled some feminists and worried psychiatrists. . . . "There's the possibility that these patients have body dysmorphic disorder, where people are obsessed with imagined ugliness," says Dr. Erik Hollander, a professor of psychiatry at the Mount Sinai School of Medicine, who is an expert on the condition.[32]

At this point, it seems like wild speculation that many women who undergo genital cosmetic surgery could meet the criteria for BDD diagnosis. Currently there are no statistics to support such a claim. According to the psychiatric literature, however, the vast majority of people with BDD who actually seek surgery want rhinoplasty, not genital surgery or other cutting-edge or controversial procedures. Whatever the reality, the term has become a readily available code for any surgery or patient considered crazy or disturbing.

In the most sensationalized stories, BDD patients are described as dangerous to others. For instance, one journalist suggests that "some even became aggressive towards doctors. . . . For the surgeons' own sake they need to protect who they are operating on."[33] Many articles mention the "one or two murders" cited in the psychiatric literature, which are raised as evidence of the volatility of people with BDD. The murder that is usually recited in the psychiatric literature and in journalistic accounts is that of Dr. Vazquez Anon in Spain. The patient, an unhappy male rhinoplasty patient who had blamed his cosmetic surgeon and had shot the doctor and his two nurses, was described by Ulrich Hinderer in *Aesthetic Plastic Surgery* in 1977 as having a pathological personality and an unhappy home life.[34] Hinderer considered the case a warning to plastic surgeons everywhere to look out for disturbed patients. That patient was never diagnosed with Body Dysmorphic Disorder, but the media's portrayal of people with BDD utilizes highly stereotypical images of the mentally ill, including associating them with this patient's violent tendencies. Mental disorder makes good newspaper and magazine copy, because "the entertainment sector of the media utilizes the precise stereotypes held by the public to describe mentally ill characters in dramatic presentations. These portrayals emphasize stereotypically bizarre symptoms of mental illness such as unpredictability [and] dangerousness."[35] These depictions reflect and affirm existing stereotypes about the mentally ill, and they socially problematize the rising popularity of cosmetic surgery. They may also affect people who have been diagnosed with the disorder, if David Veale, writing a review of the psychiatric literature on BDD in *Postgraduate Medical Journal*, is right that: "BDD patients generally feel misunderstood and are secretive about their symptoms because they think they will be viewed as vain or narcissistic. They may indeed be stigmatised by health professionals who view only true disfigurement as worthy of their attention or who confuse BDD with body dissatisfaction."[36]

The widespread media interest in BDD for the most part does not implicate the cosmetic surgery industry. The psychiatric perspective popularized by body image theorists and invoked in media accounts assumes that cosmetic surgery is medically and politically neutral. In the media, it is particular patients, those who appear to overuse cosmetic surgery or to use it in socially disturbing ways, who appear to be pathological. In the more precise medical usage, particular patients for whom cosmetic surgery is a solution to an individual, biologically rooted psychological problem are pathological. This view irks some feminists, for whom cosmetic surgery itself is the problem. Feminists might agree that some women might be especially vulnerable, but many feminists view all cosmetic patients as victimized to some degree. They argue that our culture is obsessed with beauty and body work to such a degree that the boundaries between pathological and normal uses of cosmetic surgery are impossible to draw. Virginia Blum asks, for instance, "How do body-image theorists reconcile their pathologization of beauty-obsessed people with their own work suggesting that the good looking profit in all respects?"[37]

Surgeons' Understandings of Body Dysmorphic Disorder

Cosmetic surgeons offer another vantage point from which to view surgery addiction and Body Dysmorphic Disorder. Surgeons often have little experience with diagnosing mental illness, and they do not usually subscribe to feminist views of beauty culture, either. But since the start of what is called "modern" cosmetic surgery in the nineteenth century (when anesthetics and sterilization techniques popularized surgery as a beauty practice), surgeons have been interested in assessing the motives and characters of their patients. They have employed psychological discourse to describe patients and to defend their profession to a wary public. As historian Sander Gilman describes, the use of rhinoplasty to transform racially or ethnically marked bodies into assimilated ones was justified on the basis of alleviating the mental suffering that such markings were perceived to cause.[38] And the early-twentieth-century surgical innovator Maxwell Maltz reportedly "not only eliminated scars and repaired damage with skin grafts, but removed 'deeper scars' as well—the 'scars of the mind.' "[39] Surgeons adopted Alfred Adler's notion of the inferiority complex to describe the mental illness of the ugly or stigmatized patient.[40] In other words, cosmetic surgery was generally touted as *good* for patients' mental health, which would otherwise be troubled by the stigma of belonging to an ethnic minority or by the stigma of ugliness.

Surgeons have made distinctions about the suitability of patients based on criteria that do not differ much from the larger social attitudes about cosmetic surgery. Kathy Davis describes cosmetic surgeons' long history of critiquing their patients, particularly about the validity of their wishes. While surgeons were uncritical of themselves and their profession, they were dismissive of patients. She writes: "Early cosmetic surgeons . . . maintained and helped construct the image of the cosmetic surgeon as a rugged, male explorer, embarking on exciting adventures in unknown territory . . . [while] some were quick to ridicule their patients as vain society women engaged in the trivial pursuit of beauty."[41] Patients were criticized for being frivolous in particularly gendered ways. They were also sometimes thought to be seriously misguided. Davis writes of Maxwell Maltz, "when a beautiful woman wants an operation on her face, he resists her request, relying on a mysterious 'sixth sense' which tells him that this is not her 'real' problem."[42]

Cosmetic surgery patients are still sometimes seen in highly gendered and classed terms as "socialites," divorcees, or rich widows who have money to burn and who don't really know what they are doing when it comes to cosmetic surgery. But at the same time, cosmetic surgeons today assert that their patients are not silly, vulnerable, or emotionally frail, but rather individuals making rational choices about what they want. Surgeons' attitudes are consistent with the ideology of lifestyle medicine, which suggests that individuals should use medical technology for beauty and lifestyle as well as health. Generally, they see women who get cosmetic surgeries, even most that get multiple procedures, as people who understand the social pressures surrounding youth and beauty and who want to improve or maintain their looks and their self-esteem.

Although cosmetic surgery and its patients are becoming more acceptable, cosmetic surgeons still have criticisms and worries about their patients' suitability. Body Dysmorphic Disorder has become a primary focus in patient screening.[43] Cosmetic surgeons have become more aware of BDD through newspaper and television reporting, articles in cosmetic surgery and dermatology research journals, panels on BDD at professional conferences, and their trade publications like *Cosmetic Surgery Today*. Some are directly solicited by psychiatrists. As Dr. Gellar, an ophthalmologist and cosmetic surgeon, described to me, "In the last couple of years, I've received two letters from local psychiatrists saying 'I'd be happy to see your patients,' soliciting for these [BDD] patients. There is more awareness about it in the past two years."

The diagnosis is now accepted in the cosmetic surgery industry, but there is still debate about its prevalence. In their effort to weigh in on public discussions about BDD, the ASAPS published a survey of its members in 2001, which indicated that they thought approximately 2 percent of prospective patients they see show signs of BDD. This is "a number consistent with the estimated percentage of BDD sufferers in the general population, but not as high as found in some studies investigating the prevalence of BDD among persons who seek cosmetic surgery."[44] The ASAPS is officially keen to educate its members about BDD, but also wants to dampen speculation that BDD is a widespread problem in cosmetic surgery. In one press release, for example, the ASAPS described BDD as a "rare psychiatric disorder," in contrast to the psychiatric accounts that describe it as common.[45] Among surgeons I interviewed, there was wide disagreement about its prevalence. Some see it as common. For instance, Dr. James, a facial plastic surgeon from Long Island, told me that he sees three to five patients *per week* whom he thinks are likely to have BDD. But others, like Dr. Michelle Copeland, a plastic surgeon in Manhattan, believe BDD is "extremely rare." In addition, some surgeons think that the medical crisis of BDD is "overblown," in the words of Dr. Carlton, a New England plastic surgeon.

Although cosmetic surgeons are being urged by psychiatrists to screen for BDD, no screening used to diagnose BDD has thus far been accepted as a standard. Phillips and Dufresne's screening questionnaire has been presented for use in dermatology and cosmetic surgery settings, but it has not been adopted industrywide.[46] Dr. Carlton described to me his experience with the test: "I used it on about fifty patients. It didn't help. I thought it was too obvious." The problem for Carlton was that prospective surgery patients know how to present themselves as good candidates. In his words: "these patients sitting in my waiting room, I've got what they want. They're not going to answer these questions. They want to have surgery. They're not going to admit they think about their nose twelve hours a day." Carlton suggests that cosmetic patients are strategic in presenting themselves to the surgeon. The ASAPS makes this argument as well. "[S]urgeons are not psychiatrists, and even the most thorough consultation cannot always identify the surgical candidate who is unsuitable for psychological reasons. Inappropriate behavior may not be manifested during the interview process; in fact, it is sometimes carefully masked."[47] People with BDD are seen as manipulative, tricking doctors into doing procedures they shouldn't do by lying about previous surgeries or by being insistent or persuasive.

Without reliable diagnostic screening, how do surgeons identify patients who have BDD? I asked surgeons if it was easy or difficult to tell if someone has Body Dysmorphic Disorder. Some felt confident that they could discern the disorder in a patient. As. Dr. McCullen put it, "You can pretty much get a sense for psychological stability." Surgeons would discover the mental health of the patient through their intuitive and interpersonal skills. They would get information through "a good interview with the patient," a feeling that something was wrong "in my gut," or even "picking up a vibe from someone." An article in *Cosmetic Surgery Times* describes this idea that one can read patients interpersonally as "a sense of intuition."[48]

While the "sixth sense" is regularly invoked in cosmetic surgery discourse, it is far from foolproof. Some surgeons suggest that BDD can be difficult to discern until it is "too late," after a patient has had surgery and remains unhappy.

There are specific flags surgeons look for, although they are not universally agreed upon. The cosmetic surgeons I interviewed listed a wide and sometimes contradictory set of signs of signs for BDD. In addition to the DSM criteria for BDD—perceiving a flaw that didn't exist (or was minor) and worrying about it excessively to the point of social or psychological impairment—they added criteria of their own. Some believe that patients who are on antidepressant medication are more likely to have BDD. Dr. Gellar, for example, said that she sends "those patients packing." Others are not so certain that antidepressants make a patient suspect, but they do look for other signs that a person is emotionally unstable. Dr. Bartholomew, an ENT, suggested that those in psychotherapy were more suspect. And Natasha, a medical tech who works in Dr. Bartholomew's office, described how BDD patients might not be "comfortable with themselves" or "know who they are." Moreover, they have unrealistic expectations of surgery. "They think it [surgery] will bring a significant improvement in the rest of life. People get disappointed if the man of their dreams walks by them [after the surgery]. It is sad. Their problem is in a different layer of life. They are looking in the wrong place." This kind of disappointment is part of BDD, according to some surgeons. Dr. Bartholomew suggested that BDD patients could be people who are "very ugly and want to be a ten." A number of the surgeons, including Dr. McCullen, suggested that BDD patients are unhappy with previous surgeries.

Although according to the psychiatric literature the rates of BDD among men and women are roughly equal (some estimates even put men slightly ahead of women), the surgeons I interviewed tended to describe BDD as a women's illness. They cited examples like Joan Rivers, Cindy Jackson (the so-called "Barbie woman"), widows, socialites, "young gorgeous women," and women who are upset "when the man they want walks by them." Like the media depictions of BDD, some surgeons also mentioned "weird tastes" that other people would find abnormal as indicative of BDD, and insisted that they would avoid doing any procedure that they thought could be perceived as weird or unusual. They specifically named Michael Jackson and the so-called Cat Lady, Jocelyn Wildenstein, as examples of people who may have BDD. They also found that people who are "oversurgeried, overprocessed," as Dr. Gellar put it, were probably BDD sufferers, and one mentioned Joan Rivers as an example of this. Excessive surgeries were often mentioned, although what constitutes "excessive" varied widely. Five surgeries, sixteen surgeries, and twenty-five surgeries were suggested as examples of how many surgeries people with BDD might have. One surgeon is quoted in *Cosmetic Surgery Times* as describing BDD patients as "having gobs and gobs—ten to fifteen to twenty—cosmetic procedures done."[49]

While what counts as an excessive number of surgeries remains vague, it is one of the most common ways that BDD is described by the media and by cosmetic surgeons. Yet many patients are having multiple and repeat cosmetic surgeries. According to the ASPS, 34 percent of cosmetic surgery patients had more than one procedure during an operation in 2004, and 40 percent of patients had had cosmetic surgery in the past.[50] For some, like Dr. Copeland, this may reflect an appropriate "packaging" of surgeries to achieve an overall aesthetic improvement. Or, as Dr. James, the facial plastic surgeon from New York, sees it, some of these people may be "hooked" on cosmetic surgery. Even so, being hooked is not the same thing, according to him, as having BDD. "A lot of people get hooked. That's not BDD. Not when they're doing different procedures. Lots of people get a rhinoplasty. They like the result, and then think about doing their lips. Then they want a chemical peel. That's just somebody bitten by the bug." There is a line to draw, then, between people with BDD and "ordinary" avid consumers of cosmetic surgery. A surgeon quoted in *Cosmetic Surgery Times* drew a similar line: "I'm excluding those with body dysmorphia disorder. I'm excluding the people who are certifiably nuts. I am talking about the ordinary people that I see who have repeat cosmetic surgery. . . . For them, looking nice and having a certain image is very important."[51]

Dr. James suggests that what accounts for the rise in the number of people having multiple surgeries is not the rise in mental illness but the rise of cosmetic surgery television shows, which have made it more socially acceptable to have surgery. "Everybody's going to do it [now]," he speculated. Because of its visibility on television, cosmetic surgery has been "taken out of the black box," he argues, and "people aren't afraid of it anymore." The surgeons I interviewed readily attributed media exposure with the recent market explosion. But some of them discount the idea that media exposure and beauty culture create pathological levels of surgery obsession. Consistent with the medical model of BDD, they consider surgery addicts to have individually specific, often biologically rooted psychological problems. These problems lead such people to have unrealistic expectations of cosmetic surgery. Dr. Geller, who is female, put it this way: "We're *all* exposed to media. Yeah, I'd like to look like Christy Brinkley but I'm realistic. . . . You have to have something wrong with you to have BDD. I don't think you can blame it on the world and not yourself."

There may be rational reasons why a person might have multiple surgeries, even on the same body part. In fact, she or he might be trying to correct an undesirable result from a previous surgery. Dr. Carlton and Dr. James both do many secondary surgeries—that is, they repeat a surgery already done by another doctor. This may account for the fact that although both of them seem to see a significant number of patients who they think have BDD, they are also wary of surgeons' assumptions that unhappy or difficult patients who want one surgery after another are showing symptoms of the disorder. As Carlton puts it, "[Other surgeons] confuse BDD patients with unhappy patients. Cosmetic surgeons will come up to me and tell me, 'I've got a patient with BDD. She is upset because she didn't like her scars,' or 'One side's different than the other, and she was furious.' That's not BDD. That's a problem with the surgery." Dr. James agrees, and also insists that the difficulty of rhinoplasty, which according to the psychiatric literature happens to be the surgery most requested by BDD sufferers, makes repeated rhinoplasties likely. "The reality is, this is the most difficult surgery. They could do a real shit job. . . . Most surgeons don't embrace a problem when it happens or try to fix it. They ignore the patient, or try to blame it on the patient. Someone who comes to me might have already had two or three surgeons who didn't know what they were doing."

It matters to surgeons whether or not a patient has BDD. At the very least, surgeons are aware that their procedures are aesthetically, if not medically, risky, and they are keen to please patients and avoid unhappy ones. Although not all surgeons speak as frankly as Dr. Gellar, the ophthalmologist who says she avoids troubled patients "like the plague," some doctors are concerned that unhappy patients will be hostile or difficult. Dr. Bartholomew, for example, said that because his practice is busy enough, he "doesn't need the trouble" of treating difficult patients. And Dr. Williams said that he thinks addicted patients "can't tolerate the margin of error" in surgery, or that they will be more unhappy with bad results than a "normal" patient. Moreover, surgeons are concerned about malpractice and see people with BDD as particularly litigious. This has become more salient since *Lynn G. v Hugo*, a widely publicized court case I describe in the next chapter, in which a prominent plastic surgeon was sued for malpractice for operating on a woman who claimed to have BDD.

The Construction of Surgery Addiction

Body Dysmorphic Disorder is a social construction that is becoming socially problematized. It is built from medical, media, legal, and other social practices as a framework for identifying and defining a problem or set of problems. This doesn't mean it isn't also a lived, embodied reality for some people. As medical accounts of body image disorder suggest, there are people who acutely suffer from obsessing about perceived flaws of the body. BDD may be a vital diagnosis for organizing medical and social understandings of their self-body relationships, and such people may welcome the identification of BDD as an official illness that can be socially recognized and treated. However, the relationship between BDD and cosmetic surgery is far from straightforward. The diagnosis is being invoked, questioned, and maintained differently by psychiatrists, cosmetic surgeons, feminists, the media, and others.

As I described in the previous chapter, for many feminists, cosmetic surgery is both a response to and a trigger for pathology: cosmetic surgeons prey upon women who have internalized patriarchal pressures about beauty and youthfulness, and women's exposure to beauty surgery renders them "surgical," ever seeking surgical perfection. The rise of BDD as a diagnosis challenges this view of cosmetic surgery, because although it buttresses the link between psychopathology and cosmetic surgery, it also biologizes the issue of surgery obsession. Psychiatrists want to bring attention to the psychic suffering of individuals who have a distinct, biologically rooted problem. They see the profession of cosmetic surgery as largely ignorant of the pathology and as catering to the pathological demands of sick people. Even though relatively few cosmetic surgery patients have actually been diagnosed with BDD, psychiatrists in the United States and Britain have suggested that all cosmetic surgery patients be screened for mental illness. Of course, the prospect of requiring cosmetic surgeons to screen for mental illness is highly controversial. Skeptics say that this would be a difficult regulation to enforce, and they point out that screening would require a standard, demonstrably effective test for BDD, which does not currently exist.

Surgeons have their own reasons for being concerned about BDD—about to what extent it exists and how to identify it. The prospect of unhappy, litigious, difficult, dangerous, or mentally ill patients is worrisome for them. Professionally, surgeons have to be responsible for protecting their own patients as well as their practices. They are also concerned about the overall perception of cosmetic surgery in the broader culture. Surgeons have benefited from the relative acceptability of cosmetic surgery and its patients, and yet it is in their interest that they do not appear to be ignoring or fostering pathology. Yet in a sense, BDD also offers an opportunity for cosmetic surgery, because the diagnosis is a way to draw lines between normal and abnormal patients and to define and make sense of problems of surgical excess. When the ethics of cosmetic surgery are unsettled, the diagnostic criteria for identifying mentally ill or problem patients might be useful for surgeons.

In addition to the scientific evidence presented by Phillips and other BDD specialists, the current sociohistorical context helps explain why BDD has become embraced as a cognitive tool, clinical diagnosis, and media buzzword. First, psychiatry has a relatively newfound ability to develop diagnostic categories that can quickly become recognizable and accepted.[52] The past thirty years have seen a significant development in the use of psychiatric drugs to treat mental suffering, an increased acceptance of psychiatric diagnoses and pharmaceutical treatment by health insurers, and the tripling of the number of official diagnoses in the DSM. Psychiatry's transformation influences the ease with which we adopt psychiatry's diagnostic terms in public discourse to define (and even stimulate) social controversies. Second, there is an unprecedented explosion in cosmetic surgery market, and for the first time we see widespread polysurgery. Third, this explosion takes place in a society which is still ambivalent about cosmetic surgery, and which lacks much normative or regulatory certainty about how much surgery is enough, and how much is too much. Fourth, there is relative silence from cosmetic surgery patients. Despite the rise of patient self-advocacy movements in recent decades, cosmetic surgery patients do not generally advocate as a group, or even identify as a group. For various reasons, many cosmetic surgery patients stay in the closet. Cosmetic surgery is often seen as personally embarrassing, and it is not a socially acceptable cause for self-advocacy. Patients often see surgeons as their allies in contests over cosmetic surgery, and have thus far let surgeons speak for them.[53] But this still leaves a certain silence in the rhetoric of cosmetic surgery, some of which is being filled by the media. Finally, there is the enormous media interest in cosmetic surgery. As Mark Tausig et al. argue, the media tend to sensationalize social problems related to mental illness.[54] In this context, BDD is operating as a lighting rod for social thinking about the problems of cosmetic surgery.

There are some reasons to find this worrisome. Despite Phillips and Dufresne's claim that over-diagnosing is always better than under-diagnosing, the prospect of over-diagnosing mental illness is also worrying. There are serious implications for women and others likely to be pathologized. Pathologizing cosmetic surgery patients has the same practical effect as pathologizing other kinds of people. They become discredited persons, as the sociologist Erving Goffman would have described them.[55] A diagnosis of mental illness—or even, as I established here, the *suspicion* of mental illness—is often taken to be the defining feature of a subject's behavior, dwarfing other possible explanations. In practical terms, this means that patients' own perspectives on cosmetic surgery may be silenced, and their complaints about the outcomes of surgery or the behavior of surgeons or their own beliefs about surgery may be dismissed. Cosmetic surgery patients are now in a double bind. As Suzanne Fraser puts it, "To be successful, candidates for surgery must have a dual outlook on the procedure. They should believe that cosmetic surgery alone can improve self-esteem, but they should not have too high expectations. Unrealistic expectations lead to disappointment, further psychological damage and even litigation. In some cases, litigation itself is posed as a possible indicator of mental illness. Where the surgeon deems the operation a success, the patient's failure to agree is pathologised."[56]

When pathologizing comes too easily, we put the burden of the industry's problems disproportionately on the psyches of individuals. This is not where most of the problems of cosmetic surgery belong. Feminists know this, but feminist critiques have often ended up engaging in an endless agency-choice debate. Psychiatrists may or may not support cosmetic surgery practices, but their focus firmly establishes the root of the problem in an individually diagnosable disorder. Surgeons privately recognize that there are problems in their own field, but they consistently resist any notion of regulation, hoping instead that their colleagues will voluntarily practice restraint. And the solution often focuses on sorting the good from the bad patients, with the former wanting the right surgeries, at the right times, and knowing how to find good surgeons, the latter pushing the envelope of normalcy in various ways. Seeking to sort out the good from the bad prospective patients may protect some people, surgeons and patients, from unhappy results, but such a strategy does not address cosmetic surgery's larger problems. Moreover, such sorting has to be seen as disciplinary, producing the model patient, the appropriate use of medical technology, and the outlines of a proper body-self relationship. One has to ask whether this industry and its culture ought to exercise such power to define body image and the body-self.

5

The Surgery Junkie as Legal Subject

When cosmetic surgery is linked to mental disorder, it becomes a social problem, raising a significant set of worries for medical decision making and the public. Possible scenarios of surgical excess and addicted or obsessed patients trouble cosmetic surgeons, psychiatrists, critics of cosmetic surgery, and others. Given the frequency of malpractice suits in American medicine, one of the social institutions where such scenarios will inevitably play out is the courtroom. Such a story unfolded in the New York State courts in recent years. A woman named Lynn G. underwent surgeries of the face, neck, breasts, abdomen, and legs, seeing her cosmetic surgeon a total of more than fifty times over six years. She later regretted the operations. In *Lynn G. v Hugo*, she claimed that her surgeon, Dr. Norman Hugo, ought to have realized that she was unreasonably obsessed with cosmetic surgery and, in fact, had Body Dysmorphic Disorder. The case raises many troubling questions, a number of which were debated in media coverage of the case. Should a patient be able to sue her surgeon for performing surgery she has elected? To what extent should a doctor question the normalcy of his or her patients' desires for multiple surgeries? Does it matter if his or her patient had been under psychiatric treatment for depression? If the patient was a surgery addict, how would that impact the medical standard of care? Whose responsibility is it to check surgical excess, and to diagnose Body Dysmorphia?

The case itself is an anticlimax: it ends in summary judgment for the defendant—prevented from going to trial—and offers few answers to the broader questions it provokes. But *Lynn G.* is interesting because, among other things, it is one of the first entrances of the surgery addict into the courtroom, indicating the potential of the diagnosis to organize legal and medical decision making about cosmetic surgery, as well as what kinds of social and media responses a court case about a cosmetic surgery addict might raise. In addition, I see the conundrums and paradoxes the case presents as shaped partly by what Foucault calls the hermeneutics of the self—the drive to establish the truth of the subject.

From the perspective of the judges and lawyers, whether or not there were triable issues in the case was the legal question at hand. But the case can be read beyond the narrow grounds on which it was decided, because the court records acknowledge broader questions about cosmetic surgeons and patients. After presenting the events of the case, I describe a range of possible constructions of the surgery addict as a legal subject that one can imagine from reading the various court opinions of *Lynn G.* I find instances where the patient might be perceived variously as a rational consumer, a narcissist, or a mentally ill victim. I see these constructions as forms of subjectivation resonant with widely held but disparate ideas about cosmetic surgery patients. The debates over the subjectivity of *Lynn G.*

in the court opinions effect a powerful interrogation of the subject that reflects the broader hermeneutics of the self of cosmetic surgery culture.

Lynn G. v Hugo

Lynn G. was a middle-aged woman living in New York City. Dr. Norman Hugo was a prominent plastic surgeon in Manhattan, chief of plastic surgery at Columbia-Presbyterian Hospital in the early 1990s, and a past president of the American Society of Plastic Surgeons. Lynn met Dr. Hugo when she was in her early forties, after she brought her daughter into his office for a rhinoplasty. Having already had some cosmetic surgery performed by other surgeons, including rhinoplasty, she saw Dr. Hugo more than fifty times over the next six years for various procedures, including periodic fat injections to the face, blepharoplasty (eyelid surgery), several liposuctions of the face, eyebrow tattooing, and skin growth removals (including the removal of lesions, skin tags, papillomas, and keratoses). Eventually, in February of 1993, Lynn G. also underwent liposuction of the abdomen, thighs, knees, and flanks as well as a bilateral mastopexy (breast lift). After reporting dissatisfaction with the results of the liposuction, Lynn G. underwent another operation nine months later, this time a full abdominoplasty, along with liposuction of the inner thighs.

Mrs. G., as she is referred to in some of the court documents, had been dissatisfied with the results of the February liposuction on her abdomen, and was also disappointed with the scarring that resulted from the abdominoplasty. In 1995, she filed a malpractice lawsuit, along with her husband who sued for lack of consortium (the loss of spousal intimacy or sexual relations as a result of her physical or psychological injuries). Mrs. G. did not claim that Dr. Hugo had performed the operations badly. All abdominoplasties carry the likelihood of permanent scarring, and she had been informed of the potential for "ugly scars." Instead, the lawsuit argued that Dr. Hugo had otherwise failed to obtain her informed consent. Physicians are required by public health law in all states to provide informed consent, although what this constitutes varies by state. This includes the imperatives both to tell patients of any possible bad outcomes of a procedure and to present alternatives to the proposed treatment. In *Lynn G. v Hugo,* two claims formed the basis of the case for lack of informed consent. First, the plaintiff claimed that no alternative to an abdominoplasty was presented to her, such as a suction-assisted lipectomy, which is a less invasive procedure. This point was a relatively straightforward matter—did Dr. Hugo tell her that there were alternatives to a full abdominoplasty, or not? This would be determined by weighing evidence presented by each side, and ultimately the court would decide in Dr. Hugo's favor.

The second claim is the focus of my interest in the case. This claim was much more controversial, intriguing, and difficult for the court and observers, and also makes the first point moot: Lynn G. was incapable of consenting no matter what the doctor did or did not tell her about the surgery, because she suffered from Body Dysmorphic Disorder, a condition that impaired her ability to make rational decisions about cosmetic surgery. Lynn G. charged that Dr. Hugo should have known that she was mentally compromised; therefore, he was negligent in not consulting with a psychiatrist, or sending her for a psychiatric consultation, before performing the surgeries. As summarized in the majority opinion of the Appellate Court by Judge Ernst Rosenberger:

Factual questions regarding informed consent are also presented by plaintiff's allegation that she suffers from a recognized mental disorder concerning body image that impaired her ability to assess the risks and benefits of cosmetic surgery, and that the defendant should have made further inquiries into her mental state before proceeding with the surgeries. Plaintiff's known history of depression, coupled with her extraordinary eagerness for surgical alteration, raises an issue of whether defendant should have sought advice from a mental health professional before performing more and more invasive procedures upon plaintiff.[1]

Dr. Hugo denied both claims, and his lawyers challenged the ability of the plaintiff to bring him to trial. In 1999, the Supreme Court of the State of New York allowed the case to go forward. In 2000, Dr. Hugo filed for a motion in the Appellate Court, First Division, for summary judgment to prevent a trial. In a three-to-two decision, he lost. He appealed the Appellate Court's decision to the New York State Court of Appeals. In 2001, after six years of litigation, the Court of Appeals unanimously granted the cosmetic surgeon summary judgment, meaning that the court determined, on the basis of affidavits and written evidence, that there were no factual issues to be determined in trial, and that it would apply applicable law instead, which it did in his favor. In essence, Hugo was victorious, and Lynn G. ended her suit.

Two opinions of the Appellate Court (the opinion in favor of the plaintiff by Judge Ernst Rosenberger and the dissent in favor of Dr. Hugo by Judge Richard Wallach) and a final opinion of the Court of Appeals (written by Judge Ciparick) together create an interesting legal treatment of the cosmetic surgery patient. To summarize the facts from all three opinions: Lynn G. had an interest in cosmetic surgery which (everyone agreed) significantly exceeded the norm. She underwent many procedures with the same surgeon. Finally, she had two surgeries that she regretted, in part because she found the results, including scars, unsatisfactory and damaging. In retrospect, she came to a realization that she ought not to have had those surgeries, and by implication perhaps even the earlier ones, because she had an excessive interest in cosmetic surgery. During some of her years of pursuing cosmetic surgery, she was also undergoing psychiatric treatment, and by all accounts, she was both depressed and overly attracted to cosmetic surgery. These points are a matter of agreement, but the case still raises a number of questions about cosmetic surgery, Body Dysmorphic Disorder, and the responsibilities of cosmetic surgery patients and physicians. The court was asked to consider what might have been made Mrs. G. incompetent to choose surgery. What might make the mental health of some cosmetic surgery patients suspect? Moreover, whose responsibility is it to determine whether a patient is mentally ill or has BDD? And what would be the responsibility of the surgeon in treating a patient who is determined to have BDD?

Judicial narratives offer two competing interpretations of the case. That the case centers on cosmetic, elective surgeries rather than surgeries determined to be medically necessary seem to have had some impact on the various judicial opinions about *Lynn G.* In one view, the physician is more responsible than he might already be for determining consent because of the lack of medical necessity for abdominoplasty and the other procedures. In his opinion on behalf of the majority of the Appellate Court, which found in favor of the plaintiff, Mrs. G., Judge Rosenberger made a particular effort to point out that the cosmetic surgery patient should be treated the same as any other patient in at least one respect. Rosenberger argued that under public health law, cosmetic surgery must be conducted with exactly the same standards of disclosure, even though the problem to be corrected may be a matter of subjective opinion. He writes that even though cosmetic surgery is elective, the patient's rights to informed consent are exactly the same as for medically indicated surgeries: "once the patient has decided that this feature is a problem that needs to be corrected, the doctor should have no less of a duty to disclose the risks of any treatment he could offer. In other words, while the patient's dissatisfaction with her body may be a matter of taste, the choice of treatments and the expected outcomes are governed by objective medical principles."[2] At the same time, he argued that because the surgery is elective, the physician has an extra responsibility to provide guidance as to the need for surgery, particularly in light of possible mental impairment on the part of the patient: "When there is no medical need for the operation and only the patient's subjective aesthetic opinion determines her view of whether surgery should be undertaken, a physician should have some responsibility to provide objective guidance to a patient whose capacity for self-assessment is clearly disordered."[3]

The majority opinion of the Appellate Court suggested that the elective nature of cosmetic surgery does not reduce the responsibility of the physician; in fact, it increases that responsibility, since there is no medical benefit or similar standard against which the risks of surgery can be calculated. This responsibility is heightened when a patient has a "disordered" capacity for self-assessment, which the majority of the Appellate Court believed to be the case in the matter of *Lynn G.*

In contrast, Judge Wallach, writing a dissenting opinion, appeared to have weighed the matter of the elective

and cosmetic nature of cosmetic surgery against the patient rather than the doctor. Here, the elective aspect of the
surgery is judicially reassigned, and on this reading, impli-
cates the patient. He opens his opinion, which is otherwise
written in straightforward legal prose, with a quote from
John Keats's *Ode on a Grecian Urn* (1819): "Beauty is
truth, [and] that is all ye need to know." Wallach continues, "Sadly the poet died young. But from our perspective
of age and time, we may feel confident that the Grecian
who crafted the urn which inspired such lofty sentiment
undoubtedly knew something else: that an unrelenting in-
volvement with self-beautification oftimes ends up at the
bottom of the well of Narcissus."[4]

In Wallach's dissenting opinion, Lynn G.'s story is, like
the story of Narcissus, a "cautionary tale." In opening his
argument with the Greek tale of Narcissus, who gazed so
obsessively at his own reflection in a pool of water, unable
to leave, that he eventually died, Judge Wallach clearly
identifies the cosmetic surgery patient, and elective beautification surgery, as different from other medical patients
and procedures. He does not explain in explicit terms the
lesson to be derived from this cautionary tale, but it is clear
that, given the unfortunate end Narcissus comes to because of his own failure to control his vanity, and given
that Wallach defends the cosmetic surgeon throughout his
opinion without exception, he places the blame for Mrs.
G.'s medical misfortune on her own vanity.

The issue of whether or not Mrs. G. was a typical or an
atypical patient was not really in dispute; both sides agreed
that she used cosmetic surgery quite a lot more than most
people. The number of surgeries she had undergone was
raised repeatedly as a point of concern, although no one ever
specified what, by contrast, the standard might be for a normal number of surgeries. Even though it is increasingly

common that doctors perform multiple procedures on a patient, in my review of media reporting on Body Dysmorphic Disorder, as well as in my interviews with cosmetic surgeons, the desire for multiple surgeries is often cited as a reason to suspect patients of having mental disorder. In the press, the *Lynn G. v Hugo* case raised a number of speculations about who might have BDD, pointing to the desire for multiple procedures as a possible factor. For example, in the *Boston Globe,* Dr. Mark Gorney, a medical director for a malpractice insurer, declares: "If she's had a rhinoplasty, a face lift, Botox, lip, a boob job—forget it. This patient is a plastoholic."[5] Lynn G. had more than these procedures, and for everyone in the court, the excessiveness of over fifty visits seemed obvious.

But interestingly, the high number of times Lynn G. visited Dr. Hugo is cited as supporting evidence for *both* points of view. The view siding with the plaintiff describes the number of times Mrs. G. saw Dr. Hugo as indicating an abnormal, obsessive, "extraordinary" interest in cosmetic surgery, thus signaling the possibility that she had a mental illness. This fact, combined with another key aspect of Lynn G.'s medical history, her psychiatric record, was presented as evidence of Mrs. G.'s Body Dysmorphic Disorder, which was retrospectively raised as a diagnosis by the plaintiff's medical experts. Mrs. G. had been seeing a psychiatrist for four years, and had been under his care when she first entered Dr. Hugo's office. Her psychiatrist, Dr. Gerald Frieman, had diagnosed her in the late 1980s with depression and prescribed Elavil and Prozac. Mrs. G. had stopped seeing Dr. Frieman in 1990, reportedly because Prozac had improved her condition, but she indicated on a questionnaire at Columbia Presbyterian Hospital that she suffered from "extreme nervousness or anxiety." Even though Mrs. G. had only ever been formally diagnosed with depression rather than BDD, the majority

opinion of the Appellate Court found the combination of
Lynn G.'s multiple surgeries and her psychiatric history—
constituted by a formal diagnosis of depression, self-reported
anxiety, and the use of antidepressants—compelling enough
to raise questions about her mental state. The large number
of times Mrs. G. had visited Dr. Hugo and the facts of her
psychiatric history were cited as evidence in affidavit by an
expert witness, a psychiatrist, as symptoms "consistent with
a form of Body Dysmorphic Disorder." On this matter, the
majority opined,

> When this [psychiatric] history is coupled with Mrs.
> G.'s extraordinary eagerness for surgical alteration—a
> nose reconstruction by a previous surgeon, followed
> by 51 visits to Dr. Hugo over a six-year period, in-
> cluding three facial liposuctions, eyelid surgery, pig-
> ment tattooed onto her eyebrows, and periodic injects
> of fat and Botox (botulism toxin) to smooth out facial
> wrinkles—it raises, at the very least, an issue as to
> whether Dr. Hugo should have sought advice from a
> mental health professional before performing more
> and more invasive procedures upon Mrs. G.[6]

In contrast, the opinions in favor of Dr. Hugo—the dissenting opinion of the Appellate Court and the unanimous
opinion of the Court of Appeals—use the number of times
Lynn G. saw the doctor to opposite effect, not to prove that
she was mentally ill, but rather to suggest that she was
a savvy consumer who deserved no pity. Judge Wallach
raises the number of times she had seen Dr. Hugo as evidence that she has a deep history with cosmetic surgery,
thus proposing that she ought to have been fully aware of
what she was getting involved with. Rather than painting
her as an out-of-control, incompetent surgery addict, he
paints a picture of her as a highly informed consumer:

From 1988 until 1993, over the course of dozens of
visits to the defendant, Mrs. G. had the opportunity to
discuss and consider all manner of procedures relat-
ing to purely cosmetic surgery, and the risks related
thereto. . . . This was not the first plastic surgeon she
had consulted, nor would it be the last. . . . It should
be noted that Mrs. G. executed a signed consent form
in connection with the abdominoplasty. Plaintiffs
have offered nothing to undermine the legal efficacy
of that declaration. Given the undisputed facts of her
deep experience with plastic surgery, this knowledge-
able consent is decisive.[7]

Later, the Court of Appeals agreed. They were unimpressed
with the argument that the number of times she saw her
surgeon could be evidence that her behavior was "consistent with a form of" BDD. According to the unanimous
decision of the Court of Appeals, this does not amount to
proof that Mrs. G. actually suffered from BDD. The fact
that her medical records from her psychiatrist were un-
available (her psychiatrist had died, and the records were
lost) did not help her case; the only evidence presented
from Mrs. G. about her psychiatric treatment was that,
according to her, Dr. Frieman told her she "was crazy" to
want plastic surgery. Judge Ciparick, writing the opinion
for the Court of Appeals, argues, "The record is otherwise
devoid of proof that plaintiff actually suffered from BDD
at the time of her surgeries, or that she was mentally incapable of understanding the alternatives and risks associated with the procedures."[8]

So the Court of Appeals rejected the plaintiff's argument that her desire for repeated cosmetic surgeries alone,
in the absence of other evidence, should have been interpreted as symptomatic of Body Dysmorphic Disorder. But

as important in this litigation as whether or not Mrs. G. actually had BDD was the question of whether or not Dr. Hugo should have acted to find out whether or not she did This raises important issues: should a cosmetic surgeon know the signs for BDD? And what exactly are the signs? Is desire for a lot of plastic surgery a clear sign of BDD? Whose responsibility is it to know about BDD and be able to diagnose it? The case raises questions far beyond what might have been decided in this case, but in one respect the Appellate Court indicated a preference. In the opinion for the plaintiff, the Appellate Court chastised Dr. Hugo for showing "an almost complete lack of curiosity about his patient's mental state."[9] Judge Rosenberger agreed with the plaintiff that the surgeon should have taken care to determine her mental capacity to choose surgery. Whatever way Hugo viewed his patient, in Rosenberger's view, he ought to have at the very least been interested in determining the status of her mental health, and ought to have investigated it.

In his defense, Dr. Hugo had claimed in his affidavit that taking an antidepressant is not a flag for a mental health problem that would complicate consent for elective surgery. Dr. Hugo also claimed that BDD was not a widely recognized disorder—that in fact, he hadn't ever even heard of it before this case. In response, Judge Rosenberger chastised the defendant for not knowing about Body Dysmorphic Disorder. That "he had never even heard of Body Dysmorphic Disorder," according to Rosenberger, "is a disturbing confession of ignorance from a doctor who said he was a professor at Columbia University's medical school teaching hospital and the chief of the plastic surgery division of its hospital, Columbia-Presbyterian, particularly since Columbia-Presbyterian had a BDD clinic when Mrs. G. was his patient. One might expect a plastic surgeon to be cognizant of an established psychiatric condition that affects body image and could impair a patient's ability to properly appraise and consent to cosmetic surgery."[10] The dissenting opinion, in contrast, treated both the allegation that the patient had BDD and the idea that the doctor ought to have known about it as unconvincing. Like Dr. Hugo, the dissent described the diagnosis as an obscure one, with Wallach pointing out in a footnote that "Throughout the vast body of American jurisprudence, this malady is fleetingly referred to in only one reported case . . . where an accused murderer suffered from a chronically obsessive fixation with his nose."[11] According to this logic, BDD is not a diagnosis that most medical professionals would know much about and therefore Hugo had no reason to be moved by concern or curiosity about it.

In the opinion of the majority of the Appellate Court, the plastic surgeon has a responsibility to try to detect whether a patient has BDD. If there is evidence that she might have the disorder, or if there are warning signals, the surgeon should consult a mental health professional. But what exactly this consultation is *for* is a matter of confusion. The dissenting opinion and the Court of Appeals stated that not only were the facts insufficient to serve as evidence for BDD but also that there was no evidence that if Dr. Hugo had insisted she seek psychiatric counseling prior to surgery, Mrs. G. would have actually listened to the advice of the psychiatrist. Judge Wallach points out that Mrs. G. had already discounted the earlier objections of her psychiatrist. Judge Rosenberger, referring directly to this aspect of Wallach's argument, counters with the assertion that the psychiatric consultation would not have been for the benefit of helping the patient make an informed decision about whether to have surgery, but for the benefit of the surgeon to make an informed decision about whether to perform it.

The dissent makes two further points in an attempt to challenge the legitimacy of the suit. First, Wallach argues that no matter whether or not the surgeon should look for BDD, or whether the patient actually has it, there is no evidence that someone with BDD cannot consent to surgery. And second, he describes the potential policy implications of mandating psychiatric referrals for cosmetic surgery patients. He protests, "The pronouncement of such a blanket rule, imposed under threat of a malpractice lawsuit if not complied with, is far beyond the competence of any court. It presents an unacceptable form of judicial legislation by creating a subclass of both surgeons and patients who would require psychiatric guidance before undertaking elective surgery."[12]

Unsurprisingly, it was the potential policy implications of the case that not only attracted the concern of the court but also drove much of the popular and media discussion about the case. When the case went to the Court of Appeals, the American Society of Plastic Surgeons filed an amicus brief on behalf of Dr. Hugo, stating that a decision in favor of the plaintiff would create an untenable precedent, burdening cosmetic surgeons with undue responsibilities and creating special obligations and barriers for cosmetic surgery physicians and patients. The brief argued, "This new requirement will not only increase the costs of elective surgery, thereby restricting access to elective surgery in general, but also unfairly single out plastic surgeons, leaving them exposed to frivolous lawsuits."[13]

Ultimately, Dr. Hugo won in the higher court. The Court of Appeals made the following judgment: first, that there was no substantial proof that Lynn G. had Body Dysmorphic Disorder; and second, that she consented to the surgeries, having been informed of the risks. As Judge Ciparick put it, "Acknowledging these risks, plaintiff executed a consent form and, in her own handwriting, indicated 'I understand' on her hospital chart."[14] The Court of Appeals found that the evidence that would compromise this consent was completely lacking. In a seven-to-zero decision, Dr. Hugo won summary judgment in his favor, effectively ending the suit.

Constructing the Cosmetic Surgery Patient

This case presents one of the first appearances of Body Dysmorphic Disorder in the courtroom, and gives BDD a central role in a malpractice drama that raises some of the more unfortunate possibilities of cosmetic surgery—scars, regret, psychological distress, the disintegration of the doctor-patient relationship, and legal feuding. The case of *Lynn G. v Hugo* paints an unhappy picture of a deeply dissatisfied patient, an unfortunate series of surgeries, and an accomplished surgeon defending his professional judgment in court. The court, while finding that the plaintiff failed to create a material issue of fact, reflects on possible policy implications of the case and sets off heated debates in the media about cosmetic surgery. The questions of whether we can really know, and how we can determine, if someone has BDD are raised in *Lynn G. v Hugo*, as are the questions of what exactly is a healthy or unhealthy cosmetic surgery patient and whose knowledge should organize our understanding of this.[15] Surgery addiction and Body Dysmorphia are not easily addressed by medicine or the courts, but rather open a Pandora's box of problems. Although the courts in this case avoided opening that box too far, below I examine how the case records, postcase commentary, and social debates about cosmetic surgery can be read to construct the obsessed or "extreme" cosmetic surgery patient in multiple and disparate ways.

In some contemporary and particularly social constructivist perspectives within sociolegal scholarship, it is important to trace how the legal subject is produced, because the law is seen as constitutive; that is, it actually creates the subjects that create the law. From this perspective, subjects are not fixed, rational, predictable authors of a law that then governs them and by which they are judged; rather, governing conceptions of rationality (and irrationality) and other aspects of subjectivity are produced and transformed through the formal actions of legal rhetoric, litigation, and precedent (and the informal effects that these have in social life). Thus part of what is decided in legal cases is who the participants actually are.[16] This perspective also sees "everyday normative orders as mutually embedded [with], or at least reciprocally reinforcing," the law.[17] This view seems especially relevant in thinking about a case like *Lynn G. v Hugo,* and more broadly about the social construction of the "extreme" cosmetic surgery patient in institutional and public life. How one interprets the cosmetic surgery patient depends partly on how she or he is linked to broader attitudes and social norms. So far, as I have implied throughout this book, the cosmetic surgery patient is not a stable figure, but a subject being produced from multiple fields, including feminist politics, television, the media, and at least two medical specialties.

Similarly, I see different possible versions of the character of the obsessed surgery patient that can be imagined in reading the records of *Lynn G. v Hugo.* One of the problems raised by the lawsuit is whether or not Lynn G. was a victim or an agent of her own destruction. Her suit aimed to have the status of her mental health clarified as mentally disordered by Body Dysmorphia. This would necessarily limit her agency. This view would have fixed her legal subjectivity as an incapacitated subject, a mentally disturbed woman, at least when it came to cosmetic surgery, who required special vigilance by doctors. It also would have deemed her a victim in need of protection and compensation by the court. Her repeated initiations of surgical body modification would represent the compulsive behavior of a person who could not be held responsible for her own actions. This view is partially consistent with some feminist and psychotherapeutic interpretations of cosmetic surgery as a highly gendered social problem. As I described in chapter 3, many feminists have argued not only that cosmetic surgery preys upon women and is inherently victimizing but also that a woman's willingness to get cosmetic surgery is a reflection of an internal pathology. To revisit Virginia Blum's depiction, the cosmetic surgery patient is comparable to the adolescent self-cutter who is diagnosed with Delicate Self-Harm Syndrome:

> They are called delicate self-cutters, most often adolescent females who cut their skin in moments of intolerable anxiety . . . the cuts can function as counterphobic responses to a sense of internal mutilation. The delicate self-cutter becomes herself the agent of a mutilation she dreads passively experiencing. Psychoanalyst Louise Kaplan observes that "a perversion, when it is successful, also preserves the social order, its institutions, the structures of family life, the mind from despair and fragmentation" (367). Like many who undergo cosmetic surgery, Kaplan's perverts experience a deep-seated shame that needs correcting and feel defiant rather than guilty about their perversion, which they nevertheless take to be a violation of the moral order.[18]

This is cosmetic surgery as self-mutilation. Judge Rosenberger's opinion renders this interpretation of Lynn G.'s surgeries a possibility. But unlike teenage cutters, who do their work on their own in secrecy, cosmetic surgery patients engage the help of highly trained medical experts who operate with the blessings of the state. Thus Rosenberger was adamant that, at the very least, Dr. Hugo ought to have been concerned to certify the state of Lynn G.'s mental health.

If someone who gets abnormal amounts of cosmetic surgery is mentally ill, then she needs to be treated with special care by her doctors. If her desires for cosmetic surgery are perverse, then indulging her would amount to medical opportunism. The view of the cosmetic surgery patient as a victim can extend far beyond Justice Rosenberger's more limited opinion to see every cosmetic surgery patient as needing psychological screening. This scenario is regularly depicted in the social problematization of Body Dysmorphic Disorder in the media. For example, from a newspaper in the U.K.: "Dr Eileen Bradbury, a leading NHS [National Health Service] health psychologist, has accused private cosmetic surgery clinics of preying on people suffering from mental health problems ranging from depression to body dysmorphic disorder—a devastating condition which causes sufferers to hate parts of their bodies. Bradbury has condemned the clinics for not carrying out proper psychological screening of their patients and for encouraging them to have unnecessary surgery by offering money-off deals and easy credit."[19] This view places suspicion on cosmetic surgeons and raises doubt about the ethics of performing "unnecessary" surgery, while raising worries about the mental health of cosmetic surgery patients.

The surgery addict as a victim of self-hatred and of uncaring surgeons is in stark contrast to another, more critical image. The surgery-obsessed can be depicted as a vain, self-desiring subject, one so consumed by self-love and so enamored with her own image that she "falls in," so to speak, to the bottom of Narcissus's well. Judge Wallach's dissenting opinion begins with this reference. The mythical Narcissus of Ovid's *Metamorphoses* to whom Wallach refers is an unusually beautiful boy, the son of a river god, who refuses the advances of many admirers. Upon seeing his own image in a pool, he falls in love with the mirror image of himself, and unable to leave, dies there. In Brookes More's English translation, Narcissus:

> loves an imagined body which contains
> no substance, for he deems the mirrored shade
> a thing of life to love. He cannot move,
> for so he marvels at himself, and lies
> with countenance unchanged, as if indeed
> a statue carved of Parian marble. . . .
> All that is lovely in himself he loves,
> and in his witless way he wants himself:
> he who approves is equally approved;
> he seeks, is sought, he burns and he is burnt.[20]

As psychoanalytic theorist Julia Kristeva puts it, this myth is the story of "the vertigo of a love with no object other than a mirage."[21] Narcissus has made the mistake of thinking that his own image is a real being. Eventually, Narcissus realizes that he loves only a mirage, and he is horrified. Still, he cannot help himself; he cannot escape his plight. According to Ovid, Narcissus has spurned many offers of love up to this point, has been unable to embrace others, and finally loves only "all that is lovely in himself." It is a sad story, but one for which, if it is to make sense in the context of Judge Wallach's opinion, Narcissus can only blame himself. We might see narcissism in mental illness—for example, in Narcissistic Personality Disorder—but Wallach seems to use it to describe more a character flaw than a sickness.

The suspicious view of the cosmetic surgery patient as narcissistic and flawed in character is actually an old, highly gendered trope that has been present throughout the modern history of cosmetic surgery. Kathy Davis notes that the surgical innovator Maxwell Maltz, for example, was regularly critical of his own female patients for being superficial. Maltz is regularly "sickened by the onslaught of wealthy society women seeking his services for trivial reasons."[22] Throughout his autobiography, "he makes disparaging remarks about these women as the 'newly rich who are only interested in finding new ways to spend their money' or 'paper-millions ladies' who have discovered that they can lose ten years."[23] This highly classed and gendered stereotype of the cosmetic surgery patient as overly vain, rich, and shallow is one reason for cosmetic surgeons' historical desire to defend themselves and to emphasize the reconstructive aspects of plastic surgery over the purely cosmetic.

The abnormally obsessive cosmetic surgery patient can be dismissed this way, as a woman who is overly vain and self-adoring. But in contrast to either the self-absorbed narcissist or the sick victim is the third and final construction that I read in this case, that of the autonomous rational subject. The very idea of informed consent depends upon a notion of the patient as a (gender-neutral) rational person. In addition, ideas of informed consent often include the notion that the patient has an active role in the consent process. As legal scholar Hayward Bouknight describes in his review of states' informed consent policies, the prevailing assumption is that "Medical associations cannot adequately police all doctors; some responsibility lies with the patients to protect themselves. Dr. Lawrence Horowitz, former director of the U.S. Senate Subcommittee on Health, stated, 'At its best, American medicine is the finest in the world. But you can't get the best by chance—you have to work at it. And often, the choices you make are more important in determining the outcome than the nature of the disease itself.' An informed medical consumer must ask questions to make informed decisions."[24] So the patient who has the right to informed consent is also a medical consumer with responsibilities to do some work in decision making. The ideology of individualism underscores this self-help attitude. According to the ASAPS, "patients seeking cosmetic surgery have the responsibility to research prospective physicians and make sure they are properly credentialed, certified by the ABPS [American Board of Plastic Surgery], with hospital privileges for the procedure being considered (even if the procedure will be performed in an office-based surgical facility). . . . Shared responsibility between patient and surgeon helps to ensure realistic expectations and satisfying surgical results."[25] Bouknight points out that the notion of informed consent reflects "one of society's highest values, individual autonomy," and emphasizes each individual's right (and thus, ability and responsibility) to make choices about his or her own embodiment.

The Court of Appeals, which had the final say in the matter of *Lynn G. v Hugo*, rejected Lynn G.'s effort to prove her irrationality, and thus determined that her state of mind was unexceptional. In this interpretation, she is not sick, incapacitated, mentally disordered, or even just hopelessly out of control of her own desire, stuck like Narcissus with her destructive self-love. Instead, when Judge Ciparick of the Court of Appeals points to the informed consent documents that Lynn G. signed, he underlines her conscious rationality. He recounts her statement, "I understand," which he points out was written "in her own handwriting." Thus we can imagine that Lynn G. knew what she was doing when she requested surgery, and gave full, unambiguous consent to her surgeon to operate. She is an individual with the same rights and responsibilities as any other cosmetic surgery patient. She is someone who made a conscious choice to undergo each surgery. She enacted her role as the informed, consenting patient. In addition, as Judge Wallach pointed out, she can be construed as a savvy, rather than naive, consumer who had every opportunity to ask questions, given the depth of her experience with cosmetic surgery.

A "Recognized" Disorder?

As legal scholars Scott Phillip and Ryken Grattet describe, when new concepts are introduced into the courtroom, the outcome is often "unsettled" judicial rhetoric, which is characterized by uncertainty and wrangling and restatements of definitions.[26] The unsettled status of BDD is reflected in the fact that the very idea of whether BDD is a recognized disorder was up for debate. In wrangling over whether Body Dysmorphic Disorder is a recognizable disorder, Judge Wallach described it as an obscure diagnosis with almost no precedent in medical law. In contrast, Rosenberger asserted its legitimacy on the basis of its "recognized," "established" psychiatric status and the fact that Columbia Presbyterian Hospital (where Dr. Hugo worked) had a clinic specifically dedicated for BDD patients. Dr. Hugo himself claimed that he had never heard of Body Dysmorphic Disorder. This claim might not actually be as outrageous as the majority in the Appellate Court thought. As I described in the last chapter, the foremost authorities on BDD, including psychiatrist Kathy Phillips, have said that BDD is under-recognized, and that even most mental health professionals—let alone cosmetic surgeons—know little about it.

Of course, the litigation itself and the press surrounding it provided occasions for the expansion of BDD's public recognizability. In media and legal coverage of the case, BDD was defined over and over again, and its legitimacy affirmed by reference to its definition in the DSM. From the *New York Observer's* coverage: "Body Dysmorphic Disorder would qualify as maximum distortion [of body image]. A recognized condition, it is listed in the American Psychiatric Association's Diagnostic and Statistical Manual of Mental Disorders."[27] Even though the Court of Appeals ultimately rejected Lynn G.'s claim, the court case provided the occasion for the repeated defining of Body Dysmorphic Disorder in public discourse. In the years since the case, BDD has received even more attention.

The case raised a good deal of public discussion about the implications of BDD for cosmetic surgery, psychiatry, and medical litigation. In their assessment of whether or not, from the perspective of malpractice lawyers, BDD can be legitimately invoked, Thomas Moore and Matthew Gaier surmised that: "The fact is, like the tobacco industry, which preys upon people's addiction to nicotine, plastic surgeons are in a position to exploit patients with psychiatric disorders. . . . If the standard of care in the profession requires either an investigation or a referral for psychiatric clearance, there is no reason that a departure from that standard should not give rise to a claim [of malpractice]."[28] But there is not yet such a standard of care for a psychiatric referral or clearance. In a 2001 press release, the ASAPS stated that "Plastic surgeons are not trained as mental health professionals. There is no foolproof method for us to differentiate sufferers from BDD from many others seeking elective cosmetic surgery."[29] Even so, Michael Riccardi, writing in the *New York Law Journal*, had announced after Justice Rosenberger's majority Appellate

Court opinion that "Surgeons must take into account their patients' psychiatric conditions in obtaining informed consent for elective surgery, a panel of the Appellate Division, First Department, decided yesterday . . . [even though] Justice Rosenberger said that the majority ruling did not impose a blanket rule, and only required the physician to take into account the known impairments of their patients before accepting their informed consent to surgery."[30]

The media coverage of the case created a public occasion for the problems of surgery addiction to be debated, and, like other media depictions of Body Dysmorphic Disorder, raised surgery addiction as a social problem. As the *Boston Globe* put it, the case "spurred much wringing of hands over whether plastic surgeons would someday be forced to get a psychiatrist's clearance for every patient."[31] The *Guardian* of London described a "global pandemic of Body Dysmorphic Disorder" in the West, and described the "complex ethical questions about whether cosmetic surgeons should do what an apparently sane patient requests, no matter how abnormal it might seem."[32] Some doctors put out press releases on their own describing their reactions to the case, and newspaper accounts raised a whole range of potential problems that the case might create for surgeons and their patients. For example, in the *New York Observer*, doctors describe the increase in lawsuits, the threat to doctor autonomy, the casting of suspicion on any patient who is on antidepressants, and the creation of a subclass of doctors and patients that require greater scrutiny than others. Three doctors are quoted:

> "Now you cannot just use your practice experience and whatever psychology you understand; now you have to start doing personality screenings in your office. Imagine the lawsuits that will occur then, where

you have to say [to a patient], 'Well, you took a standardized test that shows you have a borderline personality.' "

"You could make the argument that every single person with that outlook has a body disorder. Every
single patient could become a potential adversary."

"I feel like I'm practicing medicine in a very defensive
fashion . . . because at any point the patient who happens to have gone through a divorce two years ago and
is on an antidepressant, who wants to look better, can
turn around and say, 'I was on Prozac and you operated on me, so I was mentally incompetent.' "[33]

In the press, cosmetic surgeons and medical malpractice
attorneys were repeatedly described as "outraged" by the
case, while psychiatrists were asked to define Body Dysmorphic Disorder and elaborate on the possibilities of addiction in cosmetic surgery. The rhetoric became "shrill,"
to use legal scholar Joe Rollins's phrase.[34]

The ASPS responded to the case by filing an amicus
brief with the court protesting the possibility of forcing
changes in the way cosmetic surgeons practice. In the past
few years, the ASAPS has also developed an official response to BDD, and has announced its position on BDD in
several press releases between 2001 and 2004. Below, the
ASAPS describes its view of physician's responsibilities
to ensure informed consent, making reference to BDD
with the warning that the doctor should note if the patient
is "unreasonably bothered" by a minor flaw:

During the consultation, the plastic surgeon considers
such factors as whether: the patient has difficulty describing the desired change; the patient is unreasonably

bothered by what, objectively speaking, is a minor imperfection; the patient's friends and family are supportive or opposed to the procedure; the patient appears depressed or excessively anxious; and the patient has a history of dissatisfaction with cosmetic surgery. If the patient is seeking to repeat a procedure that has been performed in the past, the surgeon must evaluate whether sufficient improvement can be achieved to warrant another operation. Patients seeking cosmetic plastic surgery may have expectations that are not consistent with what is possible. It is in both the patient's and surgeon's best interests to bring the patient's perspectives in line with the surgeon's before any commitment to surgery. The alternative is regret instead of satisfaction after surgery.[35]

Like the ASPS, the ASAPS does not endorse what would be perceived as the more aggressive policy responses to BDD. The society does not recommend that all patients should be screened with a diagnostic test for BDD, or demand that its surgeons seek consultations with psychiatrists or refer patients for psychiatric evaluation. Its official response to BDD places the responsibility on the surgeons' shoulders, as Justice Rosenberger might have wanted, to be actively interested in their patients' mental health. But it asks only that surgeons consider these factors; it does not establish a standard measure for how much weight to give these factors or identify what actions to take. "Ultimately," stated the ASAPS in 2000, "the surgeon will use his or her best judgment, perhaps in consultation with a mental health professional, to determine whether or not a particular patient can reasonably be expected to benefit from cosmetic surgery."[36]

Surgical Excess, Subjectivation, and Agency

Lynn G. v Hugo provoked many questions from legal scholars, cosmetic surgeons, and journalists about cosmetic surgery practices. For example, what exactly counts as surgical excess? When, if ever, should either patients or surgeons be told to stop? Is the surgery addict mentally incompetent to give informed consent? What kind of person is she or he? Whose discursive knowledge should organize the public response to BDD—cosmetic surgeons, or psychiatrists? Or, alternatively, some other institution, like public health law? Who bears the responsibility for containing cosmetic surgery, or should it be contained? As this case was decided on narrower grounds, it did not put these larger questions on trial, even as it provoked them in the media and elsewhere. Even so, the case is illuminating, both in the ways that observers responded and how the records themselves contribute to interpretations of who the surgery addict is. The court opinions, postcase commentary and related discussions of BDD, malpractice, and informed consent collectively raise images of, among other things: a public health crisis, with doctors preying on the addicted; adversarial relationships between doctors and patients and the breakdown of trust in medical practice; an overreaching court creating a subclass of doctors and patients and forcing the development of unrealistic standards; a population of self-hating, victimized women, and of excessively self-loving, narcissistic women; and alternatively, informed, rational consumers who share the responsibility with doctors to use medical resources wisely.

The case answered none of the broader questions it raised about cosmetic surgery. It necessarily focused on the subjectivity of the patient, which Lynn G. herself instigated by requesting that her mental health be established for the legal record. Ironically, Lynn G. positions herself as a victim—the harmed party—because for years her cosmetic surgeon took her "at her word," to borrow Kathy Davis's term, that her desires for surgery were right and proper. This complicates the idea that the cosmetic surgery patient, at least in this case, is a rational subject with agency, free to choose. This notion of agency, which is informed by Enlightenment liberalism, is summarized by Suzanne Fraser, following the work of Nikolas Rose: "the view of the subject as autonomous and self-contained not only allows for accounts of behaviour that privilege individual decision making, action and reward, but demand it. In this way, the individual is able to claim any successes as his or her achievement alone, but must also bear responsibility for failures."[37] Although the first opinion, by Judge Rosenberger, sides with Lynn G. on this matter, the court ultimately sided with this liberal view of agency.

Whether Lynn G. was a victim or a rational agent is a hard question to answer, not only because of the unsettled status of BDD and the ambiguity of this case but also because it is what Fraser calls a "false choice."[38] The idea of cosmetic surgery patient as victim has a history of what I see as debatable notions of what constitutes proper bodies and psyches, and of essentializing and universalizing moves of logic. The patient-as-victim may also be informed by the long tradition of suspecting the mental health of the cosmetic surgery patient, no matter how many operations she has. At the same time, assertions of rational agency are also problematic. As Rose puts it, in liberal, individualist culture the person is not only free to choose but "obliged to be free" to choose."[39] This is particularly so in American medicine, where the consumer model is "empowering" people to take all manner of medical matters into their own hands, and where individuals' own knowledge about

medical decisions is often touted as a substitute for regulation. In the terms of Dr. Horowitz, it is the job of the patient to ensure her best chances for good medical care.

In this context, the case of *Lynn G.* seems to be an example of the "games of truth" to which Michel Foucault,
Gilles Deleuze, and others have objected. Many questions
that have been raised in reaction to *Lynn G.* cannot be answered in this game, which was forced not simply by the
deeply personal experience of Lynn G.'s surgeries and her
unhappiness about them but also by their historical context, to be played in the way it was, to center on the question of Lynn G.'s character. This context includes, among
other factors: the significant expansion of cosmetic surgery
as a private medical market; the rise of aggressive medical
and cosmetic surgery advertising; the long history of pathologizing women who get cosmetic surgery, and, paradoxically, the increasing willingness of doctors and patients to
undertake multiple surgeries; the rise in prominence of
and the expansion of the DSM; the official recognition of
Body Dysmorphic Disorder in the DSM; the public effort to
incorporate the psychiatric understanding of surgery addiction into the everyday practice of cosmetic medicine; and
the current available strategies for redressing medical complaints. More broadly, we can add the conception of agency
increasingly expressed by, and expected of, patients; the
cultural imperatives of seeing oneself as a "self to be
fixed," both physically and psychologically; and the prominence of the interior self, whether it be healthy or sick,
in our culture in general, and in our interpretations of
cosmetic surgery more specifically. To borrow Timothy
O'Leary's phrase from his reading of Foucault, such factors
may constitute "the field of possible practices . . . [and] the
processes through which dominant solutions emerged."[40]
This reading forces us to see cosmetic surgery and its

problems as social matters, rather than as wholly personal ones. It also brings us to a different kind of ethical question than is usually raised in cosmetic surgery. In Foucault's terms, we have to ask, "how much does it cost" persons to speak the truth about themselves?[41] The costs for Lynn G. of establishing her diagnosis for the legal record, even if she had won her suit, were significant. She cast doubts on her mental wellness. Her every desire for bodily transformation was painted with the same brush; her body-self relationship was fixed in a diagnosis; her body itself, already transformed, was rendered evidence for pathology. Claiming any such label forces "individuals back on themselves and fixes them to their own identities 'in a constraining way.' "[42] Of course, there may be many ways in which Lynn G. would have been empowered, had she won. But as I see it, the personal and political costs of this contest are high. Neither the ethics of cosmetic surgery nor the standards of care were established in this suit, but the onus of cosmetic surgery's complicated issues was placed squarely on the psyche of the patient.

6

The Self and the Limits of Interiority

The analysis I have presented here challenges various attempts to understand and identify the subjectivity of the cosmetic surgery patient. I argue that the hermeneutics of the self around which cosmetic surgery culture turns are themselves expressions of power relations. In this chapter, I address the implications of this view for thinking about agency and the self in cosmetic surgery. I take up the problem of how we can know the self at all in the wake of the poststructural critique of subjectivity that I have applied here. I argue that we must decenter the subject of cosmetic surgery, without losing grasp on how central she is to its power relations. I offer my own story of having cosmetic surgery, in order to explore how we might approach the self of cosmetic surgery under these difficult epistemological circumstances.

Techniques of the Self

The culture of cosmetic surgery can be understood as dominated by what Michel Foucault termed the

hermeneutics of the self, the culturally driven, institutionally supported need to interrogate, interpret, and assert the
truth of individual subjectivity. The interrogation might
use an interview questionnaire, a diagnostic screening, an
application, a biographical history or medical records, or be
less direct than any of these instances, but in all of these
cases the subject of cosmetic surgery—the patient or potential patient—is called upon to tell or otherwise reveal
the truth of her self.

Alongside the discursive work of others, then, the subject of cosmetic surgery is produced by the work of the self.
But the self is not isolated from, or indifferent to, the social
pressures surrounding her. For example, as Debra Gimlin
suggests, cosmetic surgery patients use narrative strategies
to make sense of their decisions to have cosmetic surgeries
and to render them more intelligible to others. The meanings of cosmetic surgery get articulated in anticipation of
the listener's response, as Judith Butler might put it, and in
a larger context of the field of the possible.[1] Thus the inter-
action between the external and internal meanings of cosmetic surgery shapes the subject's attempt to account for
herself. The strategic aspect of narration, which is surely
not limited to the interview encounter but extends to many
aspects of the lived experience of cosmetic surgery, points
to the intersubjectivity of even the most personal of cosmetic surgery's meanings. This insight troubles attempts
to find the truth of cosmetic surgery in any account of
the self; one cannot take a person at her word without
considering how that word is inherently communicative,
social, and intersubjective, and indeed how the self is. The
self narrating the meanings of cosmetic surgery, the self
whose identity it is that cosmetic surgery affirms or expresses, or the self who is or wants to be deemed normal (or
in Lynn G.'s case, pathological) is a self that is acting and

reacting in the field of possibilities, of intelligibility, already in play.

Michel Foucault described modern Western society— what he called "disciplinary" society—as marked by the secular confession, in which we continually seek to discover the truth of the individual. Foucault saw the confession, originating in Christian ritual, as the model for Western techniques of self-constitution in psychiatry, medicine, and other institutions. In *The History of Sexuality Vol. I*, for example, Foucault described how scientific knowledge of sexuality aimed both to discover the truth of individual sexuality and to assert the significance of that sexuality as a primary marker of identity. The purpose of sexology, and later, psychoanalysis, was to uncover the repressed or hidden character of an individual's sexuality as a way to understand and treat the individual's self. Similarly, the purpose of treatment in the asylum was to render the madman aware of his unreason, to "recognize himself in a world of judgment that enveloped him on all sides," as Foucault writes in *Madness and Civilization*.[2] Ultimately, to be cured, the mentally ill person required self-renunciation; she must see herself as mentally ill in order to be so no longer.

The confession is thus a technique of the self; it is used not only in formal interactions with psychiatrists and other experts but also in the self's relation with itself. Foucault addressed techniques of the self in his later work, including the third volume of *The History of Sexuality*. Modern techniques of the self demand a person's accounting for herself, in terms of who she is, her individual identity. The self is continually pressed to make herself intelligible through identifying with normative forms of subjectivity, habit, and disposition. The self is thus not a given, and in contemporary life, perhaps less so than ever.

Anthony Giddens has noted the increasingly elective character of our identities; he has pointed to the breakdown of traditional markers of identity, to the diasporic conditions of global life, and to the rise of consumer culture as factors in shaping us as people who must now create our own sense of self. Increasingly, we find ourselves engaging in identity work in order to establish who we are. For Giddens, identity work contains democratic possibilities for the self. For Foucault, however, identity work is not elective, but compulsory. We are forced to identify with something, and more important, *as* something, some category of identity that is determined outside of us. In the modern era these categories have unfolded through the knowledge/ power of institutions, particularly the closed institutions of the prison and the asylum. In Gilles Deleuze's reading, what we are increasingly seeing in postmodern life are "forms of free-floating control" that influence our self-constitutions.[3] Control society, as Deleuze calls it, has an increasingly open reach, influencing us to "continuously change from one moment to the other." In this society, "one is never finished with anything."[4] One's self is not ever established for good, but must be continually expressed and reconstituted.

Instead of seeing them as Giddens does, optimistically, Foucault views techniques of subjectivation as deeply worrying. Although they are so natural to us that we are usually unaware of them, they are expressions not of freedom but of unfreedom, because we are forced to see ourselves and identify ourselves in normative ways, and according to fields of intelligibility already laid out. And as Deleuze would point out, we are never able to stop, while the fields keep changing. In the terms I have outlined here, we are asked to continually make ourselves cosmetically well, to be coded as healthy and proper, as well as to be surgically transformed. We are faced with new categories of psychic pathology while pressured with new technologies of self-expression. We are asked to be authentic to who we really are, even though who that might be is being constantly narrated. Even so, one of Foucault's important insights is that the processes of subjectivation, which create us as seemingly stable subjects, are not forced on us without our participation. Here, agency and structure cannot be separated. Suzanne Fraser suggests that "the cultural subject, reconsidered, does not exercise an internalised or possessed agency; rather, he or she is produced through those forms of agency available in culture at any given moment."[5] When I express my agency through cosmetic surgery, I find myself becoming a cosmetic surgery patient, a category whose meanings I did not myself create. The agency I experience is culturally scripted. And yet agency does not disappear: I am not forced to choose cosmetic surgery, because rejecting cosmetic surgery is also possible. We must rethink agency, but we cannot do away with it altogether.

Similarly, we must displace the subject as the center of our analysis, but we cannot do away with her altogether. She is not the origin of meaning, but she is not absent from it either. The status of subjectivity as unfixed and culturally produced renders it an unreliable source of foundational meaning, but at the same time the self is part of the production of its meanings. This view of subjectivity demands a different approach to understanding cosmetic surgery than is undertaken in the discourses I have examined. It requires us not only to abandon the quest to discover the truth of the cosmetic surgery subject as if it were fixed or foundational but also to try to comprehend the forces that create her subjectivity. It demands the decentering of the subject without losing grasp of the centrality of subjectivity in the relations of cosmetic surgery. This is a daunting challenge, both epistemologically and personally. How might we understand the selves of cosmetic surgery differently?

Judith Butler takes up the problem of how to know and narrate the self in the wake of poststructural critiques of subjectivity in *Giving an Account of Oneself*. As the title suggests, the decentered subject renders problematic not only accounting for others but even accounting for oneself. She writes, "When the 'I' seeks to give an account of itself, it can start with itself, but it will find that this self is already implicated in a social temporality that exceeds its own capacities for narration; indeed, when the 'I' seeks to give an account of itself, an account that must include the conditions of its own emergence, it must, as a matter of necessity, become social theorist."[6] This is a difficult proposition, but one that I want to take up.

In much of the remainder of this chapter, I use this approach to critically examine my own autoethnographic account of cosmetic surgery. Autoethnography is "a reflexive variant of the field research qualitative tradition whereby the researcher and subject are one."[7] For me, this meant becoming a cosmetic surgery patient. The autoethnographic method is, of course, aligned more with art than science, even more than the other methods I have employed in this book. It can display "multiple layers of consciousness, connecting the personal to the cultural."[8] It renders more transparent the situatedness of the researcher, and demands reflexivity. But even in autobiographical accounts of the self, subjectivity is not only revealed but also produced. My own narrative of undergoing cosmetic surgery, then, cannot be taken at its word. Instead, it should be understood as an instance of self-constitution that demands critique.

An Autoethnographic
Account of Cosmetic Surgery

In January 2005, in the midst of writing this book, I had my own cosmetic surgery. I was already immersed in the world of cosmetic surgery as a researcher, but the minute I decided to have surgery myself, I became a prospective patient. This changed my experiences in talking to surgeons and patients; reading Web sites, numerous books, and articles about cosmetic surgery; and visiting clinics. I became less neutral in my interactions with surgeons. For instance, their opinions about my face, which had been regularly offered to me even as an interviewer and not a patient, mattered more. I became more aware of my face, and my nose—the part of me I had decided to transform—than ever. And so did the noses and faces of others. I read the beauty magazines I found in waiting rooms differently. I began to think not only representationally about how cosmetic surgery is sold but also more instrumentally about what is being sold, what the technology does and creates. What can be done, and to what degree of success? And my interactions with cosmetic surgery patients changed. When I revealed my intention to have surgery myself (and later, the fact of having been a patient), both people I interviewed and those I met informally became considerably more chatty, without exception. I sensed that they immediately felt less defensive. With what they perceived as a more empathetic audience, they were more frank about the pitfalls of cosmetic surgery as well as their excitement about it.

In fact, having spent considerable time in cosmetic surgery clinics, I had already felt sympathy for the women and men I encountered there. Most of them seemed to be enthusiastic about their surgeries and the results they achieved, with the exception of those who were still in bandages, who were generally miserable. Some were thinking of having another surgery at some point. But they did not seem to be the crazy junkies that one might expect from media accounts, nor did they seem to be the self-hating victims depicted in some of the more high-handed feminist descriptions. They did not intrigue me so much as their social circumstances did. Although they seemed recognizable, almost ordinary, to me, the world they were immersed in seemed less so. Their world was filled with social tensions, scrutiny, and advice that each of them had to negotiate. With magazines, advertisements, television, and media accounts presenting strong opinions about cosmetic surgery, and family, friends, and colleagues debating each of theirs in particular, they seemed to be surrounded on all sides with conflict. When I became a patient, so was I.

In choosing my own cosmetic surgery, I thought more deeply about feminist assertions that one who undergoes it is mutilating the body or will become addicted. As a professor who regularly teaches Women's Studies students, and as a writer who engages with feminist theory, I knew that my surgery would be read through a politicized lens. I considered the reactions of my students, colleagues, and peers. I did not go for a radical, norm-breaking surgery, as Kathryn Pauly Morgan would have liked. Neither did I get a surgery that corrected some very unsightly, stigmatized feature. Instead, I got a surgery that was highly normalizing and (in my estimation) unnecessary: a rhinoplasty that straightened, changed, and made more "ideal" my somewhat unremarkable nose. I was initially motivated by a desire to put myself into the role of patient, but I was also attracted to the idea that I could be more beautiful, my deep training in critiques of heteronormativity notwithstanding. Virginia Blum's description of the desire to invent

the body—not simply fix it, but sculpt it—aptly describes
my aims, although without the self-hatred, suffering, and
pathology that she insists are inextricably tied to cosmetic
surgery. I did not dislike my nose very much. I was not suffering. I considered myself a good-looking person who,
through surgery, could be made better looking. My embrace of a heteronormative ideal of beauty caused many of
my friends, students, and colleagues some discomfort.

My choice was made easier by the fact that I had
banged up my nose skiing the year before. The accident did
not change my appearance much; in fact, the change in my
profile was hard, if not impossible, to see. I had always had
a bump on the bridge of my nose, and the skiing incident,
I thought, might have exacerbated it slightly, although
I wasn't sure. Conceptually, the incident underlined the
plasticity of my nose, or, in the terms of phenomenologist
Drew Leder, made it dys-appear. Looking at it in the mirror, I wondered, was it changed? Or had it always looked
like this? Could it be different? Should it be? I wasn't
deeply concerned, and I didn't even mention the incident
to the cosmetic surgeons who inspected my nose. Only one
out of the five I consulted, the one I chose, asked whether I
had ever injured it. But the skiing incident turned out to be
much more significant than I initially thought: the surgeon
and the case manager of the clinic suggested that it made me
eligible for insurance coverage, even though we all knew
that the surgery was never intended to be reconstructive but
cosmetic, intended not to repair the nose to what it had been
but to reshape it entirely, from bridge to tip. It turns out that
surgeons regularly help people find ways to get insurance
coverage. They look for deviated septa in patients who want
rhinoplasty; they check the eyesight as part of blepharoplasty. This is well known in the cosmetic surgery world.
A patient even suggested to me that I was "lucky" I had

broken my nose, because my insurance covered half of the surgery, which cost over eight thousand dollars. Although they are beyond my purposes here, the ethical problems of this kind of logic, and of my own use of medical resources, are worth thinking seriously about.

I had feelings of class mobility as I shopped for a surgeon, even though at the start I wasn't sure I could afford cosmetic surgery. According to her personal narrative, Virginia Blum's mother had taken her to a cosmetic surgeon when she was a teenager. As sad as her story turns out to be, it is not a universal but a class-marked one. Having spent much of my youth in a poor area of rural Ohio, I was never exposed to cosmetic surgery as a young person, or much lifestyle medicine in general, and I found myself struck by the many ways, small and large, that medical care can be different for people with the means I now had—not only health insurance but some money of my own, and living and traveling in the places I do. For example, on a visit to England I went to Harley Street Clinic in one of London's poshest areas. I found fashionably decorated waiting rooms, people serving coffee and tea to the patients, and hushed and respectful tones of voice from the nurses and staff, including the nurse who interviewed me. Another clinic was in Englewood, a fancy town in New Jersey, just over the bridge from Manhattan. The doctor there, an otolaryngologist, is touted as one of New York's "Best Doctors" in various lists regularly published in the media. His practice is entirely committed to cosmetic rhinoplasty, a field in which he is considered a pioneer, and his name and face appear in countless magazine articles and news programs. Another doctor was located in Great Neck, Long Island, the town immortalized as a haven for the rich in F. Scott Fitzgerald's *The Great Gatsby*. The clinic I eventually chose was on the Upper East Side of Manhattan, across town from where I lived. There, I had the doors held open for me by doormen, sat in a waiting room decorated with original art, and consulted with the cosmetic surgeon on different terms than I ever had before with a doctor.

As I looked for a surgeon, I felt that I was understood as a person who was not desperate or in need of benevolence, as I have in other medical circumstances, but a little like a consumer shopping for something special and expensive. Although I did not escape unpleasantries, they were different from those I'd experienced in other medical settings. I was keenly aware of the electivity of this medical treatment: I was able to worry about a cosmetic aspect of my body rather than its very survival, its subsistence, or its health. I would be receiving medical care in high-tech, accredited facilities, with proper anesthetics and pain management, with screening for overall health, with a surgeon who had been on the faculty of a medical school. Many people who could use such resources as a matter of life and death do not get access to them. And I had much more control over choosing my doctor and my surgery, the timing and the place, than I would under different circumstances. In this sense, cosmetic surgery expressed a more leisurely approach to medical care than I have had during much of my life, and that other people have in different class and health circumstances. In this sense, I felt privileged, rather than victimized.

That is not to say that the experience was wholly pleasant. Far from it. I did not enjoy subjecting my face to intense scrutiny. All but one of the five surgeons I consulted were ready to pathologize what I thought was an unremarkable—not perfect, but hardly terrible—nose. One, an ear, nose, and throat specialist originally from Central Europe, said, "Your nose is fine. It has character; you shouldn't change it." I felt glad that in his view my nose was fine; and yet I also felt vain and silly for inquiring about changing it, perhaps because he spoke in an avuncular tone. He said that he would do the surgery if I "really wanted" it, giving me the feeling that he would be indulging me. The others, however, insisted that my nose needed to be changed. Three of these four did not see any sign of trauma, but they did see a clear case for cosmetic surgery. They also offered treatment for other body parts. From my notes after seeing the doctor on Long Island:

> *Me:* I was thinking about the bump on my nose, getting a straighter nose. But I don't want a turned-up nose. Nothing obvious.
>
> *Dr. J:* You need a smaller nose with more definition at the tip. Not turned up, but refined. You could get a chin implant, too. It's something to think about. Your profile could be more balanced.
>
> *Me:* Just my nose. I don't want anything implanted.
>
> *Dr. J:* It's often the case that we suggest a chin implant with a rhinoplasty, because we're looking at the whole profile. But it's just something to think about. Your chin is not bad.
>
> *Me: (shaking my head)* I don't want anything implanted.

I found these kinds of suggestions offensive. Despite the fact that I had offered my face up for such scrutiny, they hurt my feelings.

The fifth surgeon was a man in his late sixties who treated me both paternalistically and kindly. I chose him not for his personality but because he had performed more than two thousand rhinoplasties, and I thought experience was vital for my safety and my looks. He was likeable, matter-of-fact, and arrogant about his role as a beauty doctor. More than anyone, he disliked my nose. His view, from my notes just before I went into surgery:

Dr. W. comes in very briefly. He speaks as if he is reassuring me but is a little impatient when I ask questions.

Me: "What are you going to do?"
Him: "Straighten out the bump, refine the tip, make
it look nice. Your nose is wrong for your face;
we're going to fix that."

After the surgery, he told me that inside my nose was a
"mess," and confirmed his suspicion that I had fractured it
skiing the year before. (I should point out that the surgeon
fractured it again, as a planned part of the operation.) He
would have disliked my nose in any case, of course, because it was "wrong for my face." Although it was dis-
agreeable to hear someone describe my nose as "wrong," I
also found this reassuring. Although I did not want other
parts of me pathologized, his willingness to see my nose
this way also represented his affirmation of what would
otherwise be a silly or vain request.

Generally, the responses to my desire for rhinoplasty
can be categorized in one of two ways: either I was psychologically normal and my nose was flawed, or my nose was
normal and I was psychologically or morally unwell. The
surgeons, with one exception, saw my nose as flawed and
needing to be fixed. But the pathologized status of my nose
rendered my desire for cosmetic surgery reasonable, and
thus my psyche was perceived as healthy and proper.
(Some surgeons I consulted also screened me psychologically, usually informally. In one case, I was given a survey
that included psychological questions. All of them asked
me to define what might be a good result. Some also asked
if I had ever been on antidepressants, or been depressed. All
of them found me to be a "good candidate," even the one
who thought I didn't need a nose job.) Conversely, most of

my friends and colleagues saw my nose as fine. One said, like the first surgeon, "it gives you character." For them, my interest in changing it raised worries of victimization, pathology, or vanity. Some said that if my nose had been uglier, they may have understood my decision more. Several suggested that I had been seduced by spending too much time in cosmetic surgery clinics.

Although I should have expected these reactions, given the analysis of cosmetic surgery I had been outlining, I experienced them not only as academic matters but also as personal. What might have been the response I was looking for? Perhaps I had hoped that my desire to change my nose, and my curiosity about undergoing cosmetic surgery myself, would be affirmed without the pathologization of either my nose or my psyche. Something like, "Your nose is fine, but it's also fine to change it" is perhaps the response that would have pleased me. In only one case did I receive this kind of sentiment. My transgendered friend Paisley Currah saw my desire for surgery as something akin to his own: both of us, he said, should do whatever we want with our bodies. In his queer view, we are both performing gender acts (mine more conventional, no doubt), both embracing medical technologies to do so, and both unsettling people in the process. For him, this is a matter of rights.

The contradictions and pressures surrounding cosmetic surgery were not always about me, individually. I describe in my notes a conversation I had with Andrea, the office manager, while I was waiting to go in for surgery.

I asked her if he'd been doing a lot of rhinoplasties lately. She said: "breasts." Then we had a conversation about silicone. "We use it here," she said. "It looks better than saline. It stays softer." She went on to discuss how common it is for women to get "huge" breasts that are "inappropriate for their size," including her sister-in-law who has a tiny body but went in for [size] DD implants. Then she mentioned the Cat Lady and Michael Jackson. "Those doctors shouldn't be practicing."

Andrea's criticisms of her sister-in-law, and her mention of famous surgery junkies, were by now to me familiar. But suddenly I found this rhetoric more disconcerting. We were surrounded by fashion magazines depicting surgically modified celebrities. Brochures advertising Botox and breast implants were on the table. We were in a cosmetic surgery clinic, and I was about to undergo a permanent, face-altering operation. The incongruity between her critique of women like her sister-in-law who get too much cosmetic surgery and the setting of the clinic was striking. Later, I found myself looking at *Elle* magazine. From my notes:

> I flipped through an *Elle*, and all I noticed were the noses. Nose after nose was straight. They don't all have perfect noses, though—Sarah Jessica Parker's, for instance, is not typical. Madonna, by the way, seems to have a perfectly straight nose, from what I can tell from the Versace ads.

I had never thought so much about noses before I decided to get a rhinoplasty. Between my own growing awareness of my nose and its upcoming transformation, and of other people's views of my nose, upon which their opinions of my psyche seemed to turn, I had become nose-focused. I could imagine how others might become breast-focused, as perhaps Andrea's sister-in-law did. So much of this, I thought, lands on the shoulders of the patient: she must not be a junkie, but she should recognize how much her body needs improvement.

The physical experience of the surgery began with preparation. After over an hour of waiting (the surgeon was behind that day), I entered the examining room. I changed into a surgical robe, and waited again. I was cold and a little nervous. The anesthesiologist entered and introduced himself. He asked me questions about any medicines I might be taking. After he left, a nurse came in and took me to the operating room. I was surprised to hear a radio playing pop music. I remember nothing of the surgery except the IV and the countdown to anesthetized oblivion. (Ten, nine, eight.) Upon awaking I was lying alone in a recovery room, and began to cry from the pain.

> I am taken to the recovery room—a dark room with two metal beds separated by a curtain. I sleep but as I am waking up I feel pain. I start to cry. The nurse comes in and says, "Don't do that, you'll hyperventilate." I beg her to give me something for the pain. "Normally we want you to just take Extra Strength Tylenol," she says. I beg her again. "I can't deal with this pain. You have to give me something." She relents and tells me she'll give my sister [in the waiting room] four pills of Tylenol with codeine, but not to take them until I get home. She helps me dress and then I meet Jennifer in the waiting room. When the nurse isn't looking I pop one of the tablets.

Later, when I looked in the mirror, I felt worse: my face was not only heavily bandaged but very swollen and bruised. I was barely recognizable. I worried about my nose; what would it look like? Mostly I just wanted the pain to stop. With pain medication and some help from friends, I returned home and stayed inside for several days, except for the follow-up visit the next day to have the cotton plugs pulled out of my nostrils, which hurt quite a bit.

On the day of my follow-up appointment, I met another woman in the clinic wearing my "outfit," as my sister Jennifer called it—black eyes and nose bandages. I asked her a question, and her husband answered:

> *Me:* Had a pretty bad night?
> *Him:* She didn't sleep well at all. It was awful. I was thinking of doing it myself, but after this, no way. They act like it's going to be so easy. They don't tell you it's going to be like this. It's awful.
> *Me:* Yeah. It's hell.

But during the next few days, the swelling and pain reduced dramatically. Within a few days I went outside; within two weeks the bruising disappeared, although I wore a small bandage on my nose for several more weeks.

I remained nose-focused throughout the entire healing processes, which took more than six months. It turns out that cosmetic surgery is a practice of educated guesswork. It is unpredictable. It creates scars, swelling, bleeding, and other effects that vary from person to person, surgery to surgery. And the flesh has uncontrollable qualities: it will bleed even after the bandages are taken off, it will swell with changes in the weather, and it will reshape itself in directions that are or are not desired. Eventually, I judged my rhinoplasty to be pretty successful. I did not get a "perfect" nose, even in the view of my surgeon, but I like the result. By my own measure, my whole face looks different, and better.

After the surgery, I was asked to explain, and defend, my surgery a great deal. My students, who immediately noticed the bandage on my nose at the start of our seminar called "The Body, Self and Society," were aghast at the idea that someone they saw as a feminist would have cosmetic surgery. I gave them a story similar to the one here.

They openly debated my surgery, sometimes in the third person. Some of them wanted to defend me against suspicions of vanity or false consciousness. One student said, "She only did it because she was writing a book." Another wanted to label my surgery entirely reconstructive: "She did hurt her nose, so it doesn't count." When I pointed out to them that I elected a surgery that changed my appearance cosmetically, and that I quite liked the result, they had to ponder the contradiction, as they saw it, between my character and my actions. Many of my friends and acquaintances were also horrified, and produced many objections, of both the moral and psychotherapeutic kind. One person whom I had only known for a brief while suggested that this decision "spoke badly of my character," while a few others wondered if I would become addicted. Some were simply embarrassed for me. From my notes:

> [My friend] tells me to not announce my cosmetic surgery to others. He wants me to be in the closet. [Another friend] is glad to be able to tell people about my broken nose from skiing—it "justified" the surgery to others and makes it less embarrassing. But she says *I* can't really use it as an excuse, since I hadn't known it was broken. I don't deny that I did it for cosmetic reasons. I don't need an excuse.

Although I claim in my notes that I didn't want to use the skiing story, I did use it on occasion. Walking around the streets of New York City afterward with a bandage on my face, I provoked many curious stares and some questions. Although I felt I owed my students and friends a more complex and honest response, with strangers I sometimes employed the "broken nose" story when I did not want to engage in a prolonged philosophical debate. The skiing accident thus became a narrative resource for explaining my surgery to others, one which I mostly resisted employing but knew would be available if I wanted it.

Since my nose has healed, and I have grown accustomed to my new face, the fleshly aspects of my experience have waned in significance. My nose is largely "absent" from my consciousness, as Drew Leder would put it. However, the fact of having cosmetic surgery in my biography—its implications for who I feel that I am—remains significant. I still feel as if I have to account for myself as a person who has made this choice, and from the perspective of some, who lives in a body that is not naturally given.

The Limits of Understanding the Self

Or so this is how I narrate my story. My autoethnographic account, as any personal narrative, tries to establish authority over the meaning of my cosmetic surgery on the basis of my own subjective perspective. It is honest, but it is also inevitably strategic, in the sense that I want to be understood. This is the first of four limits of knowing and explaining the self that Judith Butler outlines in *Giving an Account of Oneself.* This account is an address; it is therefore shaped by the questions, or expected questions, of those to whom it is addressed. Butler writes, "I begin my story of myself only in the face of a 'you' who asks me to give an account."[9] My narrative here is addressed most directly to readers, who will receive it through the lens of their own ethical frameworks and politics. More broadly, my narrative is addressed to the figures who write about cosmetic surgery, to the discourses that generate its meanings, to the broader culture that codes cosmetic surgery as having particular significance. It is addressed to the forces, some I can identify and others I cannot, which seem to demand explanation of any cosmetic surgery.

But this aspect of my account also reflects the inter-subjective character of my cosmetic surgery experience. The narration I undertook to make sense of my surgery to myself and others as it was happening was influenced by, and responded to, the many people who participated in creating discussion about what my surgery means. The doctors to whom I presented myself as a prospective patient expected a certain set of attitudes about myself and my body. Andrea, the woman who worked in the clinic, was only one of many people who were pro-cosmetic surgery but were ready to identify its junkies and fools. The media and the advertisements I read urged me to transform myself, to constantly improve, and presented images of cosmetic surgery that were saturated with heteronormative promise. My students, my friends, and a few of the strangers who stared at me on the street asked for explanations, and many of them offered strong opinions that implicated me in one way or another. The cosmetic surgery world is fraught with social tension, and undergoing cosmetic surgery is not an individual project, but one that is shaped by the symbolic interactions one has with multiple others, both people and discourses, who are keen to define its meanings.

Second, my attempt to be intelligible belies the fact that there is always what Butler calls a "non-narrativizable" aspect to one's experience. While my cosmetic surgery experience is hardly unique, there are aspects of it that are entirely unique because they are rooted in my own body. That uniqueness, the aspect of my experience that is entirely my own, is compromised when translated into the more substitutable (and thus intelligible) categories of understanding. For Butler, "There is a bodily referent here, a condition of me that I can point to, but that I cannot narrate precisely. . . . The stories do not capture the body to which they refer. Even the history of this body is not fully narratable."[10] I do not experience cosmetic surgery in fully translatable terms; and yet in communicating with others, I am expected to employ methods of description that make sense to others. In doing so, I comply with already scripted codes of meaning that are set out before me. I address what are established as generic aspects of cosmetic surgery, and the issues that are already raised as significant: the pain, the beauty norms, the political debates, and the doctor-patient relationship, among others. What is lost in this narrative, I cannot say, as Butler is pointing out.

This problem is all the more poignant when the bodily experience one is trying to describe is so politicized. The third limit Butler describes is that my self-narration is shaped by the norms that discipline me. As Butler puts it, these are "norms that facilitate my telling about myself but that I do not author and that render me substitutable at the very moment that I seek to establish the history of my singularity."[11] Personal experiences of cosmetic surgery are significantly influenced by the mechanisms we now use to inscribe interior meanings onto them, and such experiences will be translated to individual selves and to the social world in recognizable templates of norms, diagnoses, and social truths. In telling my story, both here and in my daily experience of being a cosmetic surgery patient, I am being categorized according to norms and pathologies of which I am constantly being made aware, but of which I am never fully conscious. I can attempt to identify some of them: My narrative points to the influence of beauty culture and gender norms, for example as suggested by the presence of *Elle* magazine, Botox advertisements, and Versace ads. It shows a wrestling with the political debates about cosmetic surgery, both conceptually and interpersonally, with my friends and students. It suggests the influence of doctors, their ability to accept or reject my cosmetic desires, and to judge the quality of my body image. It shows the specter of pathology haunting my interactions with doctors, who are screening me, as well as with others who make distinctions between good patients and bad. There are broader effects of disciplinary culture, too, which I am aware of but do not fully grasp, that shape my gender, race, and class and otherwise influence my habits and dispositions.

These disciplinary effects include, fourth, the fixing of my subjectivity. I offer myself as a fixed "I" who can explain myself, and who speaks of having intentionality and agency. But although I am expected to define my actions with reference to an "I" that is stable and foundational, I am actually being produced "in media res, when many things have already taken place to make me and my story possible in language."[12] Butler continues, "I am always recuperating, reconstructing, and I am left to fictionalize and fabulate origins I cannot know. In the making of the story, I create myself in new form, instituting a narrative 'I' that is superadded to the 'I' whose past life I seek to tell."[13]

It may be philosophically difficult to accept the idea that we are not fixed, but rather fluid and being created and creating ourselves in the process of living, but it is not difficult for me to see my own experience that way. I call myself a cosmetic surgery patient, but this identity has no meaning outside its continual creation by the interactions between myself, others, and the social world. It is an identity that is produced as the cosmetic surgery is happening, as it is planned and undertaken and narrated. But the fluid character of this subjectivity, which I myself experience, is belied as I explain myself. The fixing of my subjectivity happens, then, both in the discourses that are pressed to define the cosmetic surgery patient as having one kind of interiority or another and in my own self-narration. The self of cosmetic surgery is continually co-constituted by the self and others, but stories of selves mask this temporal and ontological complexity.

Given these limitations, my narrative cannot authoritatively account for me, my identity as a cosmetic surgery patient, or my subjectivity. That is not simply because, in a psychoanalytic framework, I am not fully aware of my desires and fears but also because, as Butler shows, the very attempt to account is infused with intersubjective and social meaning. The perspectival shift of becoming a cosmetic surgery patient underscored this for me. From the viewpoint of researchers, feminists, doctors, the media, and others interested in cosmetic surgery, either a patient's body or her interiority, or both, are the line of focus. She is subject to their interrogation, and some truth of her self will help explain cosmetic surgery and its apparent problems. But my viewpoint became considerably different. As a cosmetic surgery patient I did not discover some internal truth that was isolated from the social interactions surrounding me. My line of focus was not wholly, or even mostly, toward myself or my interior. Although for a time I looked in the mirror more often, what I mostly experienced was a perspectival shift which allowed me to see something outside myself, but which implicated me. I saw those looking at me, and negotiated the multiple and contradictory truths that I seemed to represent.

Ethical Concerns

The critique of cosmetic surgery I have presented here is really an epistemological challenge. I have not critiqued cosmetic surgery per se, but rather our ways of understanding it, whether they be for or against. For some, this will seem to be a politically or ethically unsatisfying way of looking at the subject. When so much is at stake—the bodies of millions of women, and now men—many wish to have practical ideas of how to view it. Should we be for, or against? How should we live with cosmetic technologies? How should we deal with the bioethical problems of cosmetic surgery? If cosmetic surgery itself is acceptable, what should be the limit? How might we develop its boundaries?

There are not, in my view, easy answers to these questions, and I have purposely sidestepped them. My project, while considerably different from previous attempts to critique cosmetic surgery, also has ethical urgency. To summarize, I have argued that, first, we must consider the cosmetic surgery patient as a cultural production, one that is created in the process of becoming a patient. The meaning of the cosmetic surgery patient is being produced by various actors and forces: by televisual and other media representations; by cosmetic medicine and its ideology of cosmetic wellness; by psychiatry, with its ready diagnosis for problem cosmetic surgery patients; by feminism and other knowledges that struggle over who the patient is, and by selves who participate in cosmetic surgery. The interrelation of these and other actors is discursively shaping who the cosmetic surgery patient is, inscribing the meanings of the practice not only on the body but also on the psyche. It is important to understand these processes of inscription because, as political theorist John Ransom puts it, "Only when we comprehend the forces that make us up as individuals will we be able to respond to the overflow of activities aimed at governing the individual."[14] Therefore, second, we must respond critically to the processes of subjectivation, because the power relations of cosmetic surgery, including the consumer sell of the practices, depend upon them. Third, we must consider the politics of our pursuit of the cosmetic surgery patient's subjectivity, rather than simply the content. We need to consider not only how she responds to a question on a diagnostic screening, or in an interview, but also the fact that she has no choice but to account for herself, and must do so in ways not entirely of her choosing. We need to consider how that account is used; I argue that it is often used as a proxy for other ways of thinking about and sorting cosmetic surgery's problems. Fourth, we must find ways to understand and respond to cosmetic surgery that do not reify the cosmetic surgery patient's subjectivity. This is epistemologically challenging, but I believe it is vital to developing a reflexive and nuanced understanding of cosmetic surgery in particular, and lifestyle medicine in general.

My argument is ethically motivated, but the perspective I have outlined here, rooted in this poststructural understanding of both the subject and power relations, raises a set of questions different from those that begin with whether we support or oppose cosmetic surgery. Such questions include: Who benefits from our intense focus on the interiority of the cosmetic surgery patient? I argue that the cosmetic surgery industry does, for a start. The industry depends upon establishing the contours of a deep psychic significance to the practice, and that very significance is then exploited in the sorting of cosmetic surgery patients. The development of Body Dysmorphic Disorder as a recognizable diagnosis initially threatened some cosmetic surgeons, but even so it is becoming an institutionally useful way of screening patients, some of whom are more difficult than others. BDD is also a way to delineate boundaries around cosmetic surgery that limit the patient more than the surgeon. Whether a certain number of surgeries counts as excessive will depend, now, primarily on the character and makeup of the patient, rather than on some external judgment of what cosmetic doctors should or should not be allowed to do. This places—or as I see it, displaces—the burden of our fears about surgical excess squarely on the shoulders of individual patients. And BDD is not incongruous with, but complimentary to, the discourse of cosmetic wellness that cosmetic surgeons want us to accept. A bad patient has one set of psychic characteristics, while a good patient will have another. In fact, the whole marketing of cosmetic surgery, from doctors' advertisements to *Extreme Makeover*, relies upon selling the idea of the deep psychic significance of cosmetic surgery.

We might also ask how effective are our identifications of, and critical responses to, the problems of cosmetic surgery. The cosmetic surgery industry needs to be critically examined. But although feminism has been the most vocal critical response to cosmetic surgery, I see feminist critiques that participate in the pathologization of cosmetic surgery patients, particularly when they universalize that pathology to all women who get cosmetic surgery, as inadvertently complicit in the power relations of cosmetic surgery. I see feminist critiques that allow the possibility of women's agency as less problematic. But to the extent that they accept the parameters of the debate over women's subjectivity, that they allow a moral dilemma to be set up on the characters and consciousness of individual women, they are inadequate to address cosmetic surgery's power relations. These power relations are not only about patriarchal beauty ideals and the medicalization of beauty. They are increasingly about the medicalization, as well as the consumerization, of body image and identity. The power relations fix and center the self and the psyche; we must be critical of this positioning of the self.

We might also ask, as Foucault would, how much it

costs a subject to tell the truth about herself under these circumstances. When we insist on the primacy of individual interiority, we set up cosmetic surgery's subjects to have to define themselves in particular ways. What do they lose or gain when they do this? When they understand and explain themselves in terms set up by the current power relations of cosmetic surgery, they often feel pressured to assert their normalcy. They might do this, as many did on *Extreme Makeover* (and as I did as a cosmetic surgery patient), by accepting a pathologizing view of their bodies. When they want to challenge the behavior of their surgeons, they have to assert not only their victimization but also their mental disorder, as Lynn G. did. There are both personal and political costs to being intelligible in such ways.

Further, we can pose the question, what is lost in the overwhelming focus on the truth of the self in cosmetic surgery? I would argue that some very practical bioethical questions that I appear to have sidestepped are actually being eclipsed by the intensity of our focus on the subject.[15] Centering the patient/subject decenters other actors: the surgeons, the psychiatrists, the technologies, the media, the ideologies, the structure of medicine. There are many critical questions to ask about how cosmetic surgery works, who governs it, and who is responsible for its boundaries. There are many interrogations we can pursue, from a variety of critical perspectives, that do not rest on interrogating the truths of cosmetic surgery patients themselves.

Finally, in the spirit of Kathy Davis, whose work on agency began with a self-reflexive critique of her own feminist thinking, we can ask questions about the ethics of our problematizing cosmetic surgery. Whom do these "games of truth" help, or harm? I argue that we need to be more attentive to the politics of our truth-telling about cosmetic surgery patients, even when those truths are generated out of critical feminist concern. We must ask in what ways our critiques are operating inside of the very power relations we seek to destabilize, and how we might better refuse those relations.

Notes

Introduction

1. Dr. McCullen's and Lydia Manderson's names have been changed, as have the names of all interviewees throughout the book, except when noted.
2. Blum, *Flesh Wounds: The Culture of Cosmetic Surgery*, 66.
3. American Society of Plastic Surgeons (cited hereafter as ASPS), press release, "10.2 Million Cosmetic Plastic Surgery Procedures in 2005," March 15, 2006.
4. Ibid.
5. Sullivan, *Cosmetic Surgery: The Cutting Edge of Commercial Medicine in America.*
6. Brooks, "Under the Knife and Proud of It: An Analysis of the Normalization of Cosmetic Surgery."
7. Davis, *Reshaping the Female Body*, 90; Gimlin, *Body Work: Beauty and Self-Image in American Culture.*
8. For a similar argument, see Gremillion, *Feeding Anorexia: Gender and Power at a Treatment Center.*
9. Davis, *Reshaping the Female Body*, 126.

1 Visible Pathology and Cosmetic Wellness

1. Gilman, *Making the Body Beautiful: A Cultural History of Aesthetic Surgery*, 27.
2. Davis, *Dubious Inequalities and Embodied Differences: Cultural Studies on Cosmetic Surgery*, 101.
3. Sullivan, " 'It's as Plain as the Nose on His Face': Michael Jackson, Modificatory Practices, and the Question of Ethics."
4. Ibid.
5. Davis, *Reshaping the Female Body*, 6.
6. Grosz, "Bodies-Cities."
7. Mamo and Fosket, "Scripting the Body: Pharmaceuticals and the (re)Making of Menstruation," 14.
8. Foucault, *Discipline and Punish: The Birth of the Prison.*
9. Foucault, *The Birth of the Clinic: An Archaeology of Medical Perception.*

10. Foucault, *The History of Sexuality, Vol. I: An Introduction.*
11. Morgan, "Women and the Knife: Cosmetic Surgery and the Colonization of Women's Bodies."
12. Deleuze, *Foucault.*
13. Ibid., 57.
14. Gilman, *Making the Body Beautiful.*
15. Sullivan, *Cosmetic Surgery.*
16. Copeland, *Change Your Looks, Change Your Life: Quick Fixes and Surgical Solutions for Looking Younger, Feeling Healthier, and Living Better,* 38.
17. Dr. Copeland agreed to be identified by name.
18. Brooks, "Under the Knife," 221.
19. American Society for Aesthetic Plastic Surgery (hereafter cited as ASAPS) press release, "Psychological Study Proves Motivations of Facelift Patients," May 2, 1997.
20. ASAPS press release, "Psychological Impact: Cosmetic Surgery Improves Quality of Life," May 2, 1997.
21. ASPS press release, "ASPS Study Reveals Tummy Tucks Remove Barrier Restricting Patients' Lifestyles," July 23, 2003.
22. ASAPS, "Psychological Impact."
23. Hughes, "Medicalized Bodies."
24. Deleuze, "Postscript to the Societies of Control," 4.
25. ASAPS press release, " 'Excessive' Cosmetic Plastic Surgery: How Much Is Too Much?" February 27, 2004.
26. Ibid.
27. Nash, *What Your Doctor Can't Tell You about Cosmetic Surgery,* 53.
28. Ibid.
29. Ganny and Collini, *Two Girlfriends Get Real about Cosmetic Surgery.*
30. ASAPS, " 'Excessive' Cosmetic Plastic Surgery."
31. Pierce, "Cosmetic Surgery of Black Skin," 383.
32. Jesitus, "Ethnic Skin: Handle with Care."
33. Leydig, "Cosmetic Changes."
34. Davis, *Dubious Inequalities and Embodied Differences,* 92.
35. Lingus, *Excesses: Eros and Culture,* 25.
36. Giddens, *Modernity and Self-Identity.*
37. Shilling, *The Body and Social Theory,* 5.
38. Turner, *Medical Power and Social Knowledge,* 236.
39. Deleuze, *Nietszche and Philosophy.*
40. Fraser, *Cosmetic Surgery, Gender, and Culture.*
41. Delueze, *Foucault,* 63.
42. Ibid.

2 *Normal Extremes: Cosmetic Surgery Television*

1. Giroux, *Disturbing Pleasures: Learning Popular Culture.*
2. Fraser, *Cosmetic Surgery, Gender, and Culture.*
3. Klein, "Judges of Characters."
4. Curnutt, "The Me-Genre: Self-Reflexivity in Reality Television," 1.
5. *Extreme Makeover* (hereafter cited as *EM*), "Participant Application," http://abc.go.com/primetime/specials/makeover/application.html.
6. *EM*, "Patient Bios," http://abc.go.com/primetime/extrememakeover/index.html.
7. Weber, "Beauty, Desire, and Anxiety: The Economy of Sameness in ABC's Extreme Makeover." Her count is for seasons 1–3, all shows available as of the time of this writing.
8. *EM*, "Patient Bios."
9. Ibid.
10. Davis, *Dubious Inequalities and Embodied Differences*, 76.
11. Weber, "Beauty, Desire, and Anxiety," 13.
12. *EM*, "Patient Bios."
13. Woodstock, "Skin Deep, Soul Deep: Mass Mediating Cosmetic Surgery in Popular Magazines, 1968–1998," 421.
14. Weber, 2006. "Beauty, Desire, and Anxiety" 14.
15. Regalado and Flint, "TV Cuts Both Ways for Plastic Surgeons and for Patients: If You Want Brad Pitt's Nose, Should a Reputable Doc Give You Dose of Reality?"
16. ASPS press release, "ASPS Expert Panel to Debate Ethical Challenges in Plastic Surgery—From TV Shows to Advertising," October 26, 2003.
17. ASPS press release, "More than 8.7 Million Cosmetic Plastic Surgery Procedures in 2003—Up 32% over 2002," March 8, 2004.
18. American Academy of Facial Plastic and Reconstructive Surgery press release, "More Americans Seeking Cosmetic Surgery: 22 Percent Increase in Procedures in 2004," March 21, 2005.
19. ASPS, "More than 8.7 Million."
20. ASPS press release, "9.2 Million Cosmetic Plastic Surgery Procedures in 2004—Up 5% Growth Paces U.S. Economy Despite Reality TV Fad," March 16, 2005.
21. ASPS press release, "Cosmetic Surgery Epidemic Not Found among Young Adults," February 28, 2005.
22. ASPS press release, "Popularity of Plastic Surgery Does Not Diminish Risks: American Society of Plastic Surgeons Leads the Specialty with Safety Initiatives," March 8, 2004.
23. American Medical Association Press Release, "AMA Passes Policy on Medicare Physician Payment Cuts, Peer Review Confidentiality/Patient Safety, Reality TV, Clinical Trials," December 6, 2004.

24. ASPS press release, "New Reality TV Programs Create Unhealthy, Unrealistic Expectations of Plastic Surgery," March 30, 2004.
25. ASPS press release, "Nip/Tuck" Misrepresents the Specialty of Plastic Surgery," July 14, 2003.
26. Advertisement, *New York*, November 1, 2004.
27. *EM*, "Patient Bios."

3   Miss World, Ms. Ugly: Feminist Debates

1. Blum, *Flesh Wounds*, 289.
2. Ibid., 53.
3. Ibid., 288.
4. Ibid., 54.
5. Ibid., 289.
6. Ibid., 284.
7. Ibid., 274.
8. Ibid., 273.
9. Ibid., 290.
10. Ensler, *The Good Body*, 36.
11. Ibid.
12. Ibid., 37–38.
13. Ibid., 70.
14. Ibid., xv.
15. Frost, "Doing Looks: Women, Appearance and Mental Health," 122.
16. Bordo, "The Body and the Reproduction of Femininity: A Feminist Appropriation of Foucault."
17. Ibid., 28.
18. Morgan, "Women and the Knife."
19. Faber, "Saint Orlan: Ritual as Violent Spectacle and Cultural Criticism," 85.
20. Orlan, "I Do Not Want to Look Like . . . ," 314.
21. Orlan, "This Is My Body, This Is My Software."
22. Orlan, "I Do Not Want to Look Like . . . ," 314.
23. Davis, *Reshaping the Female Body*, 5.
24. Ibid., 177.
25. Davis, *Dubious Inequalities and Embodied Differences*, 12.
26. Ibid.
27. Davis, *Reshaping the Female Body*, 38.
28. Ibid., 113–114.
29. Davis, *Dubious Inequalities and Embodied Differences* , 14.
30. Ibid., 79.
31. Ibid.
32. Gimlin, *Body Work*, 108.
33. Ibid., 107.
34. Ibid., 105.
35. Frost, "Doing Looks," 128–129.

36. Ancheta, "Discourse of Rules: Women Talk about Cosmetic Surgery," 143.
37. Ibid., 146.
38. Ibid., 147.
39. Ibid., 146.
40. Butler, *Bodies that Matter: On the Discursive Limits of Sex.*
41. Ancheta, "Discourse of Rules," 148.
42. Ibid., 148–149.
43. Davis, *Reshaping the Female Body*, 58.
44. Gimlin, "Rethinking the Body/Self in Cosmetic Surgery," paper presented at the "Surgical Solutions" conference, McGill University, March 2006.
45. Sullivan, "It's as Plain as the Nose on His Face."
46. Jones, "Makeover Culture: Landscapes of Cosmetic Surgery."
47. Fraser, *Cosmetic Surgery, Gender, and Culture.*
48. Fraser, "The Agent Within: Agency Repertoires in Medical Discourse on Cosmetic Surgery," 28.
49. Ibid., 32.
50. Davis, *Reshaping the Female Body*, 177.
51. Fraser, "The Agent Within," 27.
52. Frost, "Doing Looks," 118.

4 *The Medicalization of Surgery Addiction*

1. Nash, *What Your Doctor Can't Tell You about Cosmetic Surgery*, 32.
2. Ibid., 31.
3. Ibid., 37.
4. Ibid., 39.
5. Ibid., 40.
6. Ibid., 43.
7. Ibid.
8. Phillips, *The Broken Mirror: Understanding and Treating Body Dysmorphic Disorder,*
9. American Psychiatric Association (hereafter cited as APA), *Diagnostic and Statistical Manual of Mental Disorders IV-TR*, 468.
10. Ibid.
11. Conrad, "The Shifting Engines of Medicalization," 13.
12. APA, *Diagnostic and Statistical Manual of Mental Disorders IV-TR*, 468.
13. Phillips, *The Broken Mirror.*
14. Neziroglu, "Body Dysmorphic Disorder: A Common but Underdiagnosed Clinical Entity."
15. APA, *Diagnostic and Statistical Manual of Mental Disorders IV-TR*, 468.
16. Wilson and Arpey, "Body Dysmorphic Disorder: Suggestions for Detection and Treatment in a Surgical Dermatology Practice,"

1391; Dee Anna Glaser and Michael S. Kaminer, "Body Dysmorphic Disorder and the Liposuction Patient," 559.

17. Aouizerate et al., "Body Dysmorphic Disorder in a Sample of Cosmetic Surgery Patients."

18. Wilkerson, *Diagnosis: Difference: The Moral Authority of Medicine*, 16.

19. Phillips and Dufresne. "Body Dysmorphic Disorder: A Guide for Dermatologists and Cosmetic Surgeons."

20. Dufresne et al., "A Screening Questionnaire for Body Dysmorphic Disorder in a Cosmetic Dermatology Surgery Practice."

21. Ibid., 457.

22. Ibid., 458.

23. Knorr et al., "The Insatiable Cosmetic Surgery Patient."

24. Nash, *What Your Doctor Can't Tell You about Cosmetic Surgery*, 90.

25. Phillips and Dufresne, "Body Dysmorphic Disorder," 236.

26. Ibid. See also Olivardia, "Body Image Obsession in Men."

27. Conrad and Schneider, *Deviance and Medicalization: From Badness to Sickness*.

28. Tausig et al., *A Sociology of Mental Illness*, 155.

29. Ibid.

30. Ibid., 156.

31. "What Is Body Dysmorphic Disorder?" *Harvard Medical School Family Health Guide*, www.health.harvard.edu.

32. Scott, "Down There, Out-There: Women's Procedures Test Limits."

33. "Plastic Surgery for Some Leads to Depression and Even Murder," *The Age* (Sydney) April 4, 2004.

34. Hinderer, "Dr. Vazquez Anon's Last Lesson."

35. Tausig et al., *A Sociology of Mental Illness*, 133.

36. Veale, "Body Dysmorphic Disorder."

37. Blum, *Flesh Wounds*, 15.

38. Gilman, *Making the Body Beautiful*.

39. Davis, *Dubious Inequalities and Embodied Differences*, 49.

40. Gilman, *Making the Body Beautiful*.

41. Davis, *Dubious Inequalities and Embodied Differences*, 33–34.

42. Ibid., 50.

43. ASAPS press release, "ASAPS Survey: Plastic Surgeons Reject Patients with Symptoms of Body Dysmorphic Disorder (BDD)," October 23, 2001.

44. Ibid.

45. ASAPS press release, "Body Dysmorphic Disorder: Update," February 20, 2001.

46. See Castle et al., "Does Cosmetic Surgery Improve Psychosocial Well Being?"

47. ASAPS, "Excessive Cosmetic Plastic Surgery."

48. Nash, "Can Cosmetic Surgery Become Addicting?"

49. Ibid.
50. ASPS, "Statistics 2004," www.plasticsurgery.org
51. Nash, "Can Cosmetic Surgery Become Addicting?"
52. Conrad, "The Shifting Engines of Medicalization."
53. Davis, *Dubious Inequalities and Embodied Differences.*
54. Tausig et al, *A Sociology of Mental Illness.*
55. Goffman, *Stigma: Notes on the Management of Spoiled Identity.*
56. Fraser, "The Agent Within," 33.

5   The Surgery Junkie as Legal Subject

1. *Lynn G. v Hugo*, 272 A.D.2d 38 (2000), 38.
2. *Lynn G. v Hugo*, 272 A.D.2d 38 (2000), 41.
3. *Lynn G. v Hugo*, 272 A.D.2d 38 (2000), 42.
4. *Lynn G. v Hugo*, 272 A.D.2d 38 (2000), 44.
5. Barnard, "When Plastic Surgeons Should Just Say 'No.' "
6. *Lynn G. v Hugo*, 272 A.D.2d 38 (2000), 42.
7. *Lynn G. v Hugo*, 272 A.D.2d 38 (2000), 49.
8. *Lynn G. v Hugo*, 96 N.Y.2d 306 (2001), 310.
9. *Lynn G. v Hugo*, 272 A.D.2d 38 (2000), 42.
10. *Lynn G. v Hugo*, 272 A.D.2d 38 (2000), 42–43.
11. *Lynn G. v Hugo*, 272 A.D.2d 38 (2000), 47, n3.
12. *Lynn G. v Hugo*, 272 A.D.2d 38 (2000), 48–49.
13. Cited by Stashenko, "Court: Doctor Had No Evidence Woman Had Body Dysmorphic Disorder."
14. *Lynn G. v Hugo*, 96 N.Y.2d 306 (2001), 308.
15. Ultimately, the court found that the plaintiff failed to produce the kind of evidence, like psychiatric records, about her diagnosis that the court intimates it might have accepted.
16. See Hyde, *Bodies of Law.*
17. Calavita, "Blue Jeans, Rape, and the 'De-Constitutive Power of Law,' " 89.
18. Blum, *Flesh Wounds*, 287.
19. Fracassini, "Clinics Prey on Plastic Surgery Addiction."
20. Ovid, *Metamorphoses*, 337.
21. Kristeva, *Tales of Love*, 42.
22. Davis, *Dubious Inequalities and Embodied Differences*, 49.
23. Ibid., 48–49.
24. Bouknight, "Between the Scalpel and the Lie: Comparing Theories of Physician Accountability for Misrepresentations of Experience and Competence," 1516–1517.
25. ASAPS, "ASAPS Survey."
26. Phillips and Grattet, "Judicial Rhetoric, Meaning-Making, and the Institutionalization of Hate Crime Law."
27. Kaplan, "What Should Plastic Surgeons Do When Crazy Patients Demand Work?"
28. Moore and Gaier, "Update on Informed Consent, Part II."

29. ASAPS, "ASAPS Survey."
30. Riccardi, "Doctor Must Weigh Patient's Mental State; Obsession with Surgeries Could Vitiate Consent."
31. Barnard, "When Plastic Surgeons Should Just Say 'No.'"
32. Hari, "Real Lives: I'm Having My Wings Done."
33. Kaplan, "What Should Plastic Surgeons Do When Crazy Patients Demand Work?"
34. See Rollins, *Aids, Sexuality and the Law: Ironic Jurisprudence*.
35. ASAPS, "Excessive Cosmetic Plastic Surgery."
36. ASAPS, "Body Dysmorphic Disorder."
37. Fraser, "The Agent Within," 30.
38. Ibid., 32.
39. Rose, *Inventing Ourselves: Psychology, Power and Personhood*, 7.
40. O'Leary, *Foucault and the Art of Ethics*, 116.
41. Foucault, "How Much Does It Cost for Reason to Tell the Truth?"
42. O'Leary, *Foucault and the Art of Ethics*, 113.

6   The Self and the Limits of Interiority

1. Butler, *On Giving an Account of Oneself*.
2. Foucault, *Madness and Civilization*, 267.
3. Deleuze, "Postscript to the Societies of Control," 2.
4. Ibid., 3.
5. Fraser, "The Agent Within," 17.
6. Butler, *On Giving an Account of Oneself*, 8.
7. Philaretou and Allen, "Researching Sensitive Topics through Autoethnographic Means," 65.
8. Ettorre, "Gender, Older Female Bodies and Autoethnography," 535.
9. Butler, *On Giving an Account of Oneself*, 11.
10. Ibid., 38.
11. Ibid., 39.
12. Ibid.
13. Ibid.
14. Ransom, *Foucault's Discipline: The Politics of Subjectivity*.
15. For some of these ethical issues, see Parens, *Surgically Shaping Children*.

Bibliography

American Psychiatric Association, *Diagnostic and Statistical Manual of Mental Disorders IV-TR*. Washington, D.C., 2000.

Ancheta, Rebecca Wepsic. "Discourse of Rules: Women Talk about Cosmetic Surgery." In *Women's Health: Power, Technology, Inequality and Conflict in a Gendered World*, edited by Kathryn Strother Ratcliff, 143–149. Boston: Allyn and Bacon, 2002.

Aouizerate, B., H. Pujol, D. Grabot, M. Faytout, K. Suire, C. Braud, M. Auriacombe, D. Martin, J. Baudet, and J. Tignol. "Body Dysmorphic Disorder in a Sample of Cosmetic Surgery Patients." *European Psychiatry* 18 (2003): 365–368.

Associated Press. "Add a 'Voice Lift' to your Tummy Tuck." http://www.cnn.com/2004/HEALTH/19/voice.lift.ap/index.html. April 19, 2004.

Balsamo, Anne. *Technologies of the Gendered Body: Reading Cyborg Women*. Durham: Duke University Press, 1996.

Barnard, Anne. "When Plastic Surgeons Should Just Say 'No.'" *Boston Globe*, September 12, 2000, p. E3.

Blum, Virginia. *Flesh Wounds: The Culture of Cosmetic Surgery*. Berkeley: University of California Press, 2003.

Bordo, Susan. "The Body and the Reproduction of Femininity: A Feminist Appropriation of Foucault." In *Gender/Body/Knowledge*, edited by Alison Jaggar and Susan Bordo, 13–33. New Brunswick: Rutgers University Press, 1989.

Bouknight, Heyward H. "Between the Scalpel and the Lie: Comparing Theories of Physician Accountability for Misrepresentations of Experience and Competence." *Washington and Lee Law Review* 60 (2003): 1515–1560.

Brooks, Abigail. "Under the Knife and Proud of It: An Analysis of the Normalization of Cosmetic Surgery." *Critical Sociology* 30.2 (2004): 207–239.

Butler, Judith. *Bodies that Matter: On the Discursive Limits of Sex*. New York: Routledge, 1993.

———. *On Giving an Account of Oneself*. New York: Fordham University Press, 2005.

Calavita, Kitty. "Blue Jeans, Rape, and the 'De-Constitutive Power of Law.'" *Law and Society Review* 35.1 (2001): 89–117.

Castle, David, Roberta Honigman, and Katherine A. Phillips. "Does Cosmetic Surgery Improve Psychosocial Well Being?" *Medical Journal of Australia* 176 (June 17, 2002): 601–604.

Conrad, Peter. "The Shifting Engines of Medicalization." Leo Reeder Award Lecture, presented at the American Sociological Association, San Francisco, August 16, 2004.

Conrad, Peter, and Joseph Schneider. *Deviance and Medicalization: From Badness to Sickness.* Philadelphia: Temple University Press, 1992 [1980].

Copeland, Michelle. *Change Your Looks, Change Your Life: Quick Fixes and Surgical Solutions for Looking Younger, Feeling Healthier, and Living Better.* New York: Harper Collins, 2003.

Curnutt, Hugh. "The Me Genre: Self-Reflexivity in Reality Television." Paper presented at Television in Translation Conference, Massachusetts Institute of Technology, Boston, May 3, 2003.

Davis, Kathy. *Dubious Inequalities and Embodied Differences: Cultural Studies on Cosmetic Surgery.* Lanham, Md.: Rowman and Littlefield, 2003.

———. *Reshaping the Female Body.* New York: Routledge, 1995.

Deleuze, Gilles. *Foucault.* London: Continuum, 1988.

———. "Postscript to the Societies of Control." *L'Autre Journal* 1 (May 1990).

———. *Nietzsche and Philosophy.* Translated by Hugh Tomlinson. London: Athlone, 1983.

Dufresne, Raymond, Katharine Phillips, Carmela Vittoria, and Caroline Wilkel. "A Screening Questionnaire for Body Dysmorphic Disorder in a Cosmetic Dermatology Surgery Practice." *American Society for Dermatologic Surgery* 27 (2001): 457–462.

Ensler, Eve. *The Good Body.* New York: Villard Books, 2004.

Ettorre, Elizabeth. "Gender, Older Female Bodies and Autoethnography." *Women's Studies International Forum* 28.6 (2005): 535–546.

Extreme Makeover. ABC. http://abc.go.com/primetime/extrememakeover/index.html.

Faber, Alyda. "Saint Orlan: Ritual as Violent Spectacle and Cultural Criticism." *Drama Review* 46.1(2002): 85–92.

Foucault, Michel. *The Birth of the Clinic: An Archaeology of Medical Perception.* Translated by A. M. Smith Sheridan. New York: Vintage Books, 1994 [1973].

———. *Discipline and Punish: The Birth of the Prison.* Translated by Alan Sheridan. New York: Vintage, 1995 [1977].

———. *The History of Sexuality, Vol. I: An Introduction.* London: Allen Lane/Penguin Books, 1979.

———. "How Much Does It Cost for Reason to Tell the Truth?" In *Foucault Live*, edited by Sylvere Lotringer, translated by John Houston. New York: Semiotext(e), 1989.

———. *Madness and Civilization.* New York: Vintage, 1988.

Fracassini, Camillo. "Clinics Prey on Plastic Surgery Addiction." *Scotland on Sunday,* April 7, 2002, p. 5.

Fraser, Suzanne. "The Agent Within: Agency Repertoires in Medical Discourse on Cosmetic Surgery." *Australian Feminist Studies* 18.40 (2003): 27–44.

———. *Cosmetic Surgery, Gender, and Culture.* New York: Palgrave, 2003.

Frost, Liz. "Doing Looks: Women, Appearance and Mental Health." In *Women's Bodies: Discipline and Transgression,* edited by Jane Arthurs and Jean Grimshaw, 117–136. London: Cassell, 1999.

Ganny, Charlee, and Susan J. Collini. *Two Girlfriends Get Real about Cosmetic Surgery.* Los Angeles: Renaissance Books, 2004.

Giddens, Anthony. *Modernity and Self-Identity.* Cambridge: Polity, 1991.

Gilman, Sander L. *Making the Body Beautiful: A Cultural History of Aesthetic Surgery.* Princeton: Princeton University Press, 1999.

Gimlin, Debra L. *Body Work: Beauty and Self-Image in American Culture.* Berkeley: University of California Press, 2002.

———. "Rethinking the Body/Self in Cosmetic Surgery." Paper presented at the Surgical Solutions conference, McGill University, Montreal, February 2006.

Giroux, Henri. *Disturbing Pleasures: Learning Popular Culture.* New York: Routledge, 1994.

Glaser, Dee Anna, and Michael S. Kaminer. "Body Dysmorphic Disorder and the Liposuction Patient." *Dermatologic Surgery* 31 (2005): 559–561.

Goffman, Erving. *Stigma: Notes on the Management of Spoiled Identity.* New York: Simon and Schuster, 1963.

Gremillion, Helen. *Feeding Anorexia: Gender and Power at a Treatment Center.* Durham: Duke University Press, 2003.

Grosz, Elizabeth. "Bodies-Cities." In *Feminist Theory and the Body: A Reader,* edited by Janet Price and Margrit Shildrick, 381–387. New York: Routledge, 1999.

Grosz, Elizabeth. *Volatile Bodies: Toward a Corporeal Feminism.* Bloomington: Indiana University Press, 1994.

Haiken, Elizabeth. *Venus Envy: A History of Cosmetic Surgery.* Baltimore: Johns Hopkins University Press, 1997.

Hari, Johann. "Real Lives: I'm Having My Wings Done." *Guardian* (London), March 11, 2002, Section G2, p 6.

Hinderer, Ulrich T. "Dr. Vazquez Anon's Last Lesson." *Aesthetic Plastic Surgery* 2 (1977): 375–382.

Hughes, Bill. "Medicalized Bodies." In *Body, Culture, and Society: An Introduction,* edited by Philip Hancock, Bill Hughes, Elizabeth Jagger, Kevin Paterson, Rachel Russell, Emmanuelle Tulle-Winton, and Melissa Tyler, 12–28. Buckingham, U.K.: Open University Press, 2000.

Hyde, Alan. *Bodies of Law*. Princeton: Princeton University Press, 1997.

Jesitus, John. "Ethnic Skin: Handle with Care." *Cosmetic Surgery Times*, June 2004. http:www.comseticsurgerytimes.com.

Jones, Meredith. "Makeover Culture: Landscapes of Cosmetic Surgery." PhD dissertation, University of Western Sydney, 2005.

Kaplan, Renee. "What Should Plastic Surgeons Do When Crazy Patients Demand Work?" *New York Observer*, July 31, 2000, p 1.

Klein, Amanda. "Judges of Characters." *Exposed: A Journal of Our Blurring Culture*. On-line journal, http://www.realityblurred .com/exposed, 2004.

Knorr, N. J., M. T. Edgerton, and J. E. Hoopes. "The Insatiable Cosmetic Surgery Patient." *Plastic and Reconstructive Surgery* 40.3 (1967): 285–289.

Kristeva, Julia. *Tales of Love*. Translated by Leon S. Roudiez. New York: Columbia University Press, 1987.

Leydig, Kimberly. "Cosmetic Changes." *Outlook* 41.1 (Spring 2004). http://medschool.wustl.edu/~wumpa/outlook.

Lingus, Alphonso. *Excesses: Eros and Culture*. Albany: State University of New York Press, 1983.

Mamo, Laura, and Jennifer Ruth Fosket. "Scripting the Body: Pharmaceuticals and the (re)Making of Menstruation." Paper presented to the American Sociological Association, Philadelphia, 2005.

Moore, Thomas, and Matthew Gaier. "Update on Informed Consent, Part II." *New York Law Journal* (August 7, 2001): 3.

Morgan, Kathryn Pauly. "Women and the Knife: Cosmetic Surgery and the Colonization of Women's Bodies." In *The Politics of Women's Bodies*, edited by Rose Weitz, pp. 147–163. Oxford: Oxford University Press, 1998.

Nash, Joyce D. *What Your Doctor Can't Tell You about Cosmetic Surgery*. Oakland, Cal.: New Harbinger Publications, 1995.

Nash, Karen. "Can Cosmetic Surgery Become Addicting?" *Cosmetic Surgery Times*, June 1, 2004. www.cosmeticsurgerytimes.com.

Neziroglu, Fugen. "Body Dysmorphic Disorder: A Common but Underdiagnosed Clinical Entity." *Psychiatric Times* 15.1 (1998): 23.

O'Leary, Timothy. *Foucault and the Art of Ethics*. London: Continuum, 2002.

Olivardia, Roberto. "Body Image Obsession in Men." *Healthy Weight Journal*, July/August 2002.

Orlan, "I Do Not Want to Look Like . . ." In *The Body: A Reader*, edited by Mariam Fraser and Monica Greco, 312–315. London: Routledge, 2005.

———. "This Is My Body, This Is My Software." Lecture delivered in London, 1997. www.orlan.net.

Ovid. *Metamorphoses*. Translated by Brookes More. Boston: Cornhill, 1922.

Parens, Eric. *Surgically Shaping Children: Technology, Ethics and the Pursuit of Normality.* Baltimore: Johns Hopkins University Press, 2006.

Philaretou, Andreas, and Katherine Allen, "Researching Sensitive Topics through Autoethnographic Means." *Journal of Men's Studies* 14.1 (2006): 65–78.

Phillips, Katharine A. *The Broken Mirror: Understanding and Treating Body Dysmorphic Disorder.* Oxford: Oxford University Press, 1998.

Phillips, Katharine A., and Raymond G. Dufresne. "Body Dysmorphic Disorder: A Guide for Dermatologists and Cosmetic Surgeons." *American Journal of Clinical Dermatology* 1.4 (July/August 2000): 235–243.

Phillips, Scott, and Ryken Grattet. "Judicial Rhetoric, Meaning-Making, and the Institutionalization of Hate Crime Law." *Law and Society* 34.3 (2000): 567–607.

Pierce, Harry E. "Cosmetic Surgery of Black Skin." *Dermatologic Clinics* 6.3 (1988): 377–385.

Ransom, John S. *Foucault's Discipline: The Politics of Subjectivity.* Durham: Duke University Press, 1997.

Regalado, Antonio, and Joe Flint. "TV Cuts Both Ways for Plastic Surgeons and for Patients: If You Want Brad Pitt's Nose, Should a Reputable Doc Give You Dose of Reality?" *Wall Street Journal*, April 7, 2004, p. A1

Riccardi, Michael. "Doctor Must Weigh Patient's Mental State; Obsession with Surgeries Could Vitiate Consent." *New York Law Journal* (June 28, 2000): 1.

Rollins, Joe. *Aids, Sexuality and the Law: Ironic Jurisprudence.* New York: Palgrave, 2004.

Rose, Nikolas. *Inventing Ourselves: Psychology, Power and Personhood.* Cambridge: Cambridge University Press, 1996.

Scott, Gale. "Down There, Out-There: Women's Procedures Test Limits." *Crain's New York Business*, October 25, 2004.

Shilling, Chris. *The Body and Social Theory.* London: Sage, 1993.

Stashenko, Joel. "Court: Doctor Had No Evidence Woman Had Body Dysmorphic Disorder." Associated Press, June 7, 2001.

Sullivan, Deborah. *Cosmetic Surgery: The Cutting Edge of Commercial Medicine in America.* New Brunswick: Rutgers University Press, 2001.

Sullivan, Nikki. " 'It's as Plain as the Nose on His Face': Michael Jackson, Modificatory Practices, and the Question of Ethics." *SCAN: Journal of Media, Culture, Arts* 1.3 (2004). http://scan.net.au.

Tausig, Mark, Janet Michello, and Sree Subedi. *A Sociology of Mental Illness.* Upper Saddle River, N.J.: Pearson/Prentice Hall, 2004.

Turner, Bryan S. *Medical Power and Social Knowledge.* Second edition. London: Sage, 1995.

Veale, David. "Body Dysmorphic Disorder." *Postgraduate Medical Journal* 80 (2004): 67–71.

Weber, Brenda R. "Beauty, Desire, and Anxiety: The Economy of Sameness in ABC's Extreme Makeover." Paper presented at the Surgical Solutions conference, McGill University, Montreal, February 2006.

Wilkerson, Abby L. *Diagnosis: Difference: The Moral Authority of Medicine*. Ithaca: Cornell University Press, 1998.

Wilson, Joshua B., and Christopher J. Arpey. "Body Dysmorphic Disorder: Suggestions for Detection and Treatment in a Surgical Dermatology Practice." *Dermatologic Surgery* 30 (2004): 1391–1399.

Woodstock, Louise. "Skin Deep, Soul Deep: Mass Mediating Cosmetic Surgery in Popular Magazines, 1968–1998." *Communication Review* 4.3 (2001): 421–442.

Index

About the Author

VICTORIA PITTS-TAYLOR received her PhD from Brandeis University and is an associate professor of sociology at Queens College and the Graduate Center of the City University of New York. She is the author of *In the Flesh: the Cultural Politics of Body Modification* (2003), as well as many articles and book chapters on social and cultural aspects of the body, and is editor of the forthcoming *The Cultural Encyclopedia of the Body*. She has won an Advancement of the Discipline Award from the American Sociological Association.